Praise for
From the Boxing Ring to the Ashram

In this well-researched book, Deborah Charnes draws from a broad spectrum of experts for practical guidance on the full range of human experience. Everyone who wants to upgrade their mind, body and spirit—and to integrate all three into a cohesive, evolving whole—will find value in these pages.

—**Philip Goldberg,** author of *American Veda,*
The Life of Yogananda, and *Spiritual Practice for Crazy Times*

I love the way Deborah Charnes brings ancient spiritual wisdom to help anyone who is facing a modern-day issue. Her soothing words help you reconnect and trust your inner knowing, which is a relief to all those seeking peace in this chaotic world. As a naturopathic doctor and psychotherapist, I know the importance of healing both your body and your mind. The wisdom in *From the Boxing Ring to the Ashram* nourishes the mental, physical and spiritual crevices of our human experience. Thank you for this heartwarming piece of work!

—**Dr. Ameet Aggarwal,** bestselling author of
Heal Your Body, Cure Your Mind

Deborah Charnes shares a cornucopia of wisdom, carefully harvested through her keen observations of remarkable life experiences. As the life sciences advance, our appreciation and gratitude grow in recognition of the depth of knowledge of the ancients. The keys to the health of mind, body and spirit are graciously revealed within the pages of this valuable gift.

—Dr. Joseph Weiss,
Clinical Professor of Medicine, UCSD

From the Boxing Ring to the Ashram is a transformative self-help book that takes readers on a journey of healing and self-discovery. Based on twelve life lessons from twelve teachers with twelve unconventional life paths dotted with challenges along the way, this book is a great addition to our yoga literature. I highly recommend it for yoga students, yoga teachers, yoga therapists, healthcare providers and scholars who are interested in the therapeutic and spiritual benefits of yoga and yoga therapy. You'll find yourself coming back to the text time and again for deeper study and practice.

—Dr. Dilip Sarkar, FACS, DLitt (Yoga),
former Associate Professor of Surgery and past president of
the International Association of Yoga Therapists

With an upbeat, pithy style and entertaining turns of phrases, Deborah Charnes unearths sagacious advice nestled in true-life encounters with people who have penetrated the ordinary and transcended challenges to bring peace and wisdom into their lives. Their stories and the author's insights show us how we can discover our own wisdom to make life more vibrant and meaningful. Every chapter includes easy, practical tips for holistic mind/body wellness.

—Pranada Comtois, award-winning author of
Wise Love, Bhakti Shakti and *Prema Kirtan*

Worldwide, 41 percent of adults feel overly stressed on a daily basis, and stress aggravates or induces many disease states. *From the Boxing Ring to the Ashram* offers a wealth of no-cost proven tools to combat daily stressors. Best of all, they can be as enjoyable as singing, dancing and laughing out loud.

—**Dr. Madan Kataria,**
founder of the Laughter Yoga Movement

Wisdom abounds, and the teacher (the guru) shows up in many ways and forms. I love all the different voices in this book, and how each one speaks the same truths to us in their own unique way. A joy to dip into and out of for inspiration!

—**Mehtab Benton,**
originator of Gong Yoga and Gong Therapy

From my personal connection to several of the featured gurus, I can attest that Deborah Charnes has a remarkable and respectable group of wise masters. Their life lessons are critical building blocks to address so much of what's plaguing us in modern society.

—**Sridhar Silberfein,** creator and executive producer of
Bhakti Fest, Shakti Fest and Luna Sol Retreats

Deborah's gentle, graceful approach allows for much comfort and joy on our journey to high-quality health.

—**Kate Eckman,** award-winning author of
The Full Spirit Workout

From the Boxing Ring to the Ashram is one of those rare books soaked in truth and love that stays connected to science and has practical tips that can be adopted instantaneously. It is a true gem for anyone who is on a quest for healing.

—**Dr. Venkat Srinivasan,**
Internal, Integrative and Mind/Body Medicine

In *From the Boxing Ring to the Ashram*, Deborah Charnes weaves her personal learnings of life with practical steps for us to make small changes in our own lives. Dense with wisdom, quotations from her teachers, scientific studies and inspiration, this book gives us short and simple examples of how we can tune in better to our mind, body and spirit. I love how Charnes demonstrates how we become who we are. Each person we meet can be a lever for our own growth and development, changing us for the better, so we can change the lives of others. Charnes exemplifies this. Enjoy this gem of a book. Ingest it in small bites so you can savor and experience the tiny lessons for transformation.

—**Liz Lipski,** PhD, CNS, author of *Digestive Wellness*

From the Boxing Ring to the Ashram is a true gem of a book that will leave you feeling inspired and empowered. Through her insightful writing, Deborah Charnes takes us on a journey to meet wise men and women from diverse backgrounds who have dedicated their lives to helping others find light in the dark spaces of life. Their teachings, combined with Charnes's own practical tips, offer a roadmap for anyone looking to live a more fulfilling and easeful life.

What I particularly love about this book is its structure, which makes it easy to turn to whenever you need a boost of inspiration. Whether you're seeking guidance on how to manage stress, be of greater service, or access more joy in your life, *From the Boxing Ring to the Ashram* has something for everyone. This book is truly a must-read, and its transformative teachings will undoubtedly have a lasting impact on your life.

—**Dev Suroop Kaur,** Director of Empowered Sound, a collective dedicated to freedom through the voice

Deborah Charnes is the real deal. Her writing is compelling, deep and engaging, but her capacity to distill the essence of the mind/body connection is what sets her work apart.

—Julie Carmen, actor and LMFT, C-IAYT

A steady spiritual practice is crucial to feed the spirit and overcome the lower natures. Deborah Charnes shares from her personal experiences and wisdom from teachers of various lineages, practical tips on how to build and sustain simple methods to feed our soul and calm the mind.

—Visvambhar Sheth, musician

Deborah Charnes recounts her personal story of dealing with chronic pain and finding yoga and yoga therapy in *From the Boxing Ring to the Ashram*. She shares inspiration from what she calls "unlikely gurus" in practical tips that can help the reader create their own toolbox of well-being practices.

—Alejandro Chaoul,
director of The Jung Center's Mind Body Spirit Institute and author of *Tibetan Yoga for Health and Well-being*

From the
BOXING
RING
to the
ASHRAM

From the
BOXING
RING
to the
ASHRAM

*Wisdom for
Mind, Body and Spirit*

by Deborah Charnes

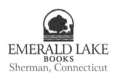

EMERALD LAKE
BOOKS
Sherman, Connecticut

Books published by Emerald Lake Books may be ordered through your favorite booksellers or by visiting emeraldlakebooks.com.

Library of Congress Cataloging-in-Publication Data
Names: Charnes, Deborah, 1958- author.
Title: From the boxing ring to the ashram : wisdom for mind, body and
  spirit / by Deborah Charnes.
Description: [Sherman, CT] : Emerald Lake Books, [2023]
Identifiers: LCCN 2023015596 (print) | LCCN 2023015597 (ebook) | ISBN
  9781945847707 (paperback) | ISBN 9781945847714 (epub)
Subjects: LCSH: Mind and body. | Well-being.
Classification: LCC BF161 .C437 2023 (print) | LCC BF161 (ebook) | DDC
  128/.2--dc23/eng/20230501
LC record available at https://lccn.loc.gov/2023015596
LC ebook record available at https://lccn.loc.gov/2023015597

Contents

Life Lessons from Unlikely Gurus

My childhood may have been happy, but it was not trouble-free. I suffered from chronic pain in my lower back and abdomen. My mom dragged me to a top orthopedic surgeon and a gastroenterologist to find answers to my multiple woes. The experts diagnosed my problems and then fortunately suggested lifestyle approaches to resolve them rather than medications or invasive interventions.

I'm thankful for those early pangs, cramping, x-rays, lab tests and even a visit to the emergency room. They led me to yoga and meditation long before mindfulness, vinyasa and hot yoga were buzzwords. Witnessing the incredible impact of simple techniques is why I later became a certified yoga therapist. I want as many people as possible to find relief for their physical and emotional afflictions through painless, inexpensive practices. That's also the reason I wrote *From the Boxing Ring to the Ashram*.

In my yoga practice, there is a special prayer to honor those who share their wisdom. There were many wise souls who transformed my life from a corporate marketing executive to a holistic coach, and I feel a deep sense of gratitude for them all. Some are swamis. Others are doctors. Then, there are gurus masquerading as students, neighbors and everyday people. Regardless, they are all teachers who found simple solutions to turn their lives around. By reading about the lessons these teachers taught me and being mindful of applying the principles to your own life, you can find greater health and happiness.

I stumbled across yoga therapy by accident—or providence. After forty years of yoga practice with five more as an instructor, I discovered a three-year yoga therapy training in an obscure location in central Florida.

Yoga therapy is not the same as yoga. It is so much more. The program I found combined my love for Ayurveda, traditional Chinese medicine, and Eastern philosophy while taking my knowledge of anatomy to another level.

Today, as a certified yoga therapist, I see myself as a cross between a physical therapist, a psychotherapist, a nutrition counselor, and a lifestyle coach. I have to know a little about everything, including when to refer clients to a primary care physician, a specialist or another complementary medicine practitioner.

My journey did not take place in the fast lane. I spent fifty years exploring the world, searching for answers, uncovering simple secrets to physical, emotional and spiritual support. It was not always easy to turn my back on long-ingrained patterns. The older they were, the more I needed to play catch up. And yet, my happiest and healthiest days came after I qualified for AARP[1] discounts.

No one should have to wait that long to find relief and healing. That is why I wrote this book. It is a collection of concrete tips for the mind, body and spirit that I gleaned from my teachers around the world.

By sharing the concepts I uncovered, I hope to spark your interest in well-being and your desire to escape the rigors of modern life.

From the Boxing Ring to the Ashram is not about total transformation or a bulldozing of your personality, belief system, or routine. Instead, these tips will help you find your true essence, accept yourself, and enhance your contentment. The approach in this book is to adopt comfortable habits that lead to a higher quality of physical, emotional and spiritual health.

Most of the suggestions you'll read here represent yoga "off the mat." It's not about sitting cross-legged or doing headstands, but bringing the peace and awareness of yoga into your everyday life. They are appropriate for everyone, anytime, anywhere and on any budget regardless of your physical abilities or limitations. You don't need to purchase any special attire, props or studio memberships. This is authentic yoga, a practice that has been whitewashed with the mass marketing of the ancient Eastern traditions and philosophy. Real yoga is about naturally finding and connecting peace of mind, body and spirit.

Big "G" Gurus and Small "g" gurus

Westerners often have a hard time wrapping their heads around the concept of a guru. American sacred music artist Adam Bauer clarified it to me this way:

> There are a lot of different ways to think about the word "guru." One definition is "that which dispels darkness," and there are many levels at which people can come into our life and help us move from darkness toward light. If we are looking for someone to be a big "G" Guru—an infallible and perfect distillation of divinity with no faults or

shadows in themselves—that is a very tall order, which is not often fulfilled in this world.

But there are many ways people can be small "g" gurus, or teachers, for us in one domain or another. We can learn from so many people and situations, even though very few people are perfect and most everyone is fallible.

In the end, I would say that one definition of the word "guru" is someone who can truly help us evolve, practically speaking, into better and more complete expressions of ourselves. And there are a lot of those people in the world, thank God.

One widely acclaimed guru, Swami Sivananda, explained in his hallmark book, *Bliss Divine*, first published in 1951, that all sages, saints, prophets and teachers had their own gurus. Acknowledging that Western culture is not as familiar with the concept, Sivananda said:

For a beginner in the spiritual path, a guru is necessary. To light a candle, you need a burning candle.[2]

I never found that one Guru. Fortunately, I found twelve small "g" gurus representing various religions, ethnicities, countries of origin, and professions.

As I introduce you to each of them, you'll discover practical, life-altering lessons to help you achieve a balanced and healthy mind, body and spirit. Each chapter is based on my personal experience with my gurus as well as my research into their lives and teachings. And you'll find their wisdom quoted throughout the chapters of this book.

My gurus are all teachers, even if they've never stood at the front of a classroom. They are all yogis, even if they've never touched a yoga mat. They all love life and their communities, and they all give 120 percent to share what they have learned. Given their commonalities, even though each chapter focuses on one life lesson and one guru, there are parallels between one chapter and another. The wisdom of my gurus steers you to better sleep, diet, interpersonal relationships, self-esteem, weight and blood sugar regulation, digestion and response to stressors. Some adversities are thankfully eased along the way: pain, stress, anxiety, depression, cognitive decline and physical deterioration.

From the Boxing Ring to the Ashram provides options to inspire you to invest in yourself by taking a fresh approach to life. Pick a chapter that feels comfortable to work on now. Then come back and add another one later.

This book is divided into three parts.

- Part I: Life Lessons for the Mind
- Part II: Life Lessons for the Body
- Part III: Life Lessons for the Spirit

Part I explores the inner workings of the brain and offers tips to help quiet the mind. Part II shifts the attention to how we can better soothe and nourish our bodies, while Part III is the icing on the cake, with chapters that contain secrets for contentment and joyful living.

Each chapter within those parts is structured the same to make it simple for you to find what you're looking for.

- I begin with a brief introduction of how I first met that chapter's guru and what life lesson they taught me.
- Then I share a bit of their background with anecdotes from the guru and insights into their

unique wisdom.

- I follow that up with further exploration of the life lesson they shared with me and how that applies to daily living.
- Next comes five quick tips and simple ideas from my guru that teach you how to begin implementing that wisdom into your life.
- Then I reveal a bit more of my experience with the topic. Since I like to understand the science behind why an approach is effective, I also share supporting studies I find interesting.
- Finally, I offer a suggestion or two for how to incorporate the guru's wisdom into your own life.

Pick and choose which life lessons you want to work on whenever it is right for you.

Since research has proven that you need forty days to change a habit, I've created a tracker you can use to track your practice over time. You can download my forty-day challenge chart at deborahcharnes.com/tracker.

While it's common to compartmentalize our issues and you may immediately be drawn to one chapter over another, I've found most of my clients need a holistic approach to addressing their emotional and physical concerns. In other words, your mind, body and spirit are all interrelated. So don't neglect taking a well-rounded approach to your well-being. Instead, find the power to live your happiest and healthiest life in the pages ahead.

I am filled with gratitude for my gurus. I spent decades searching for blueprints for well-being. Legwork, homework and travel plus a little synchronicity brought me to the best teachers for my needs. I loved every minute of winnowing these simple solutions from my inspirational sources across the globe. While I highly recommend that route, you can take a shortcut with this book.

I would love for you to achieve happiness as the Dalai Lama sees it. "Happiness is not something ready-made. It comes from your own actions." Choose those actions that bring happiness and buoy your spirit every day.

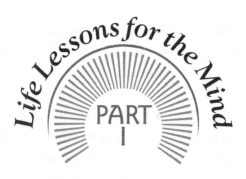

Life Lessons for the Mind

PART
I

The Brain Is Your Command Center

In our society, we tend to associate the brain with intelligence. "He's brainy." "She's got a big brain." Or "It's brain fog." Too often, we rule our lives with our mind. We give rationale and logic priority over feelings.

This is not surprising, since the brain is so complex. Many people are aware of the difference between right- and left-brain dominance. But it is much more intricate than there just being two hemispheres. It is more like a jigsaw puzzle. Each piece has a precise function and relationship with the other pieces it connects to and with the rest of our body.

At times, we can see the muscles and veins in our bodies. Outside a laboratory or hospital, we never see ligaments, nerves or the brain. Yet our intellect assures us they are all in their proper places under the surface. We take for granted the organ that differentiates us from primates and makes us each as unique as a snowflake.

Despite all my training in anatomy, as required of yoga therapists, I feel challenged when it comes to the complexities and intricate components of our master control center. We rely on our brains for reading, writing and math. We use our brains for decision-making and to create original works of art, poetry or music. Some of those mysterious parts protected by our skull rule and regulate our emotions. How we respond can make the difference between acceptance and jubilance or feelings of despair and thoughts of ending our lives.

Everyone understands the importance of eating healthy foods, whether or not they choose to. But few consider nourishing or exercising their brains. Just as we pour knowledge into ourselves, even before the time we can speak, there are ways to nurture and stimulate this organ. The three pounds of indispensable soft nervous tissue packed with eighty-six billion neurons has what seems like unlimited potential. But we need to take care of it.

Modern science supports mind over matter and the hypothesis that we can rewire our neural pathways. The no-longer-radical goal of reshaping the brain is not to help a student ace a test, but to enjoy longer, happier and healthier lives.

The life lessons in the first four chapters address the powerhouse of the brain and how its mechanisms can bring about temporary feelings of relaxation, rejuvenation and release while working behind the scenes on longer-term benefits.

While you can open the book to any chapter, sometimes it is best to start at the top—the mind.

Chapter 1: Mindfulness for Peace of Mind

*Meditation is the thread onto which
the rest of my life has been woven.*

—Shane "Christopher" Perkins

Despite my enthusiasm for a healthy lifestyle, once I hit fifty, my body was rustier and my bones were cracklier. Type 2 diabetes, a stress-aggravated disorder, was rampant in my family. With a recent prediabetes diagnosis, statistics indicated I was more at risk every year. I set aside the time and money for yoga teacher training—not to teach yoga, but for the wisdom and discipline to fuel my lifelong practice and step up the physical and stress management payoffs from Eastern traditions.

Training programs for aspiring yoga teachers are bountiful. But I wanted authenticity, discovery, enlightenment and a life-changing experience. Yandara Yoga Institute fit the bill.

A major enticement was that Yandara had its own *kirtan* band playing sacred music[3] most nights. Another draw was staying in Mexico, which I call my *segunda patria* (second homeland). I have family in Mexico City and attended college at the National Autonomous University of Mexico, the campus known for its ten-story windowless library decorated with a Juan O'Gorman mosaic masterpiece.

However, the clincher for me was reading the staff bios. I respected the yoga roots of Craig Perkins. He spent decades immersed in the Sivananda philosophy, Chinese yoga, Tibetan Buddhism, and tai chi.

Craig's son, Shane "Christopher" Perkins, was raised in that world, but he forged an awe-inspiring story of his own. His exploration of "self" shepherded him from Canada to the United States, then to India and Mexico.

The younger Perkins was my lead coach at Yandara. I learned how to teach yoga, but Christopher opened my eyes to true life lessons in living, loving, self-awareness and sharing.

The ongoing mindfulness that I learned from him was the kick in the butt I needed to redirect my future. Two years later, I was ready to chuck the corporate grind. I didn't retreat to a cave. However, I chose to redefine and rewrite my life and my career to fit with who I was at the core.

This chapter is a rare opportunity for people beyond the Yandara community to hear his kernels of wisdom. His incredible journey began as a kid who chiseled away at societal barriers to unlock an alternative pathway to love and contentment. At the end of the chapter, he offers ten techniques for a one-minute time-out to sprinkle into your daily routine.

The Teacher of Teachers: Christopher Perkins

Christopher got a serious bolt from the blue when he was an infant.

> My mother, a talented, loving, yet deeply distraught new mother and wife, left the family when I was just six months old. But life goes on.

Admittedly, Christopher's home life was atypical. Western families often emphasize educational advancement, competition, a white picket fence, color televisions, and Nintendos. This young boy grew up in a household and within a tight community where success was measured by love, happiness and a oneness with the Creator. Open-door homes he visited had vegetable gardens, prayer altars, meditation rooms, and set times of the day and night for quieting the mind and for spiritual reflection.

His father helped run a spiritual center in rural Virginia where an elderly wise man from India resided each summer. Christopher recalls:

> This humble turban-wearing guru was seen as, and is still regarded to be, a modern-day saint. With just four years of life under my Spider-Man belt, I mustered the courage to ask the swami if I could meditate with him. I was nervous, but I like to think he could see the sincerity in my eyes.

The master agreed. So the prekindergartner, like a Tibetan monk in training, got his indoctrination into true meditation. Training began, with no potty breaks or snack time. The child, just like the grown-ups, learned to sit in silence for two hours at a time.

Unsurprisingly, Christopher was the only little one among a small group of adults who was granted a formal initiation. He took to his meditations with dedication and did not balk at giving up playtime with the other tiny tots. Those practices became the backbone for his personal growth.

When Christopher was fourteen, his father completed a cloistered meditation in the backwoods of West Virginia under the guidance of John P. Milton. An ecologist, spiritual leader, and meditation master, Milton was a proponent of vision quests.[4]

Christopher's first encounter with Milton was indelible in his memory.

> I remember the day I met John. It was warm, and the sky was dotted with white, puffy clouds.
>
> My stepmother and I had just driven two hours to pick up my father. After a long and winding drive through the forest, we arrived at a primitive West Virginia cabin nestled deep in the forest. When the sounds of tires struggling against the ancient rocky terrain faded and the engine came to rest, I found myself embraced by an immense silence. I looked up and saw John sitting on the porch.
>
> Think of your favorite teddy bear becoming human, able to reassure you with just a twinkle in his eye. I didn't know much about him, but I knew he was a special person—at least to my parents.
>
> After a short, guided walk in the woods, we said our goodbyes. I'll never forget what John said to me during that first bear hug. "Whenever you're ready, we'll work together." It's like he knew that in the future I would be ready. And I was.

When Christopher turned twenty, he became John Milton's apprentice. His next few years are equally stirring and surreal, traveling through the wintry Himalayan mountains, sitting near-naked in a cave for extended periods.

He feels that decision was the single most important moment in his life. He spent three years of intense training that makes a backwoods wilderness weekend look like a Disney vacation.

I was being taught to handle the answers to the most important questions. At the end of those three years, I had no more questions. I felt completeness, simple and free, saturated in a deep knowing and peace.

After living as an itinerant ascetic, Christopher had no marketable job skills, nor a place to live. As if it were providence, John told him about some rustically developed land he owned on the southern tip of the Baja peninsula in Mexico. The property could use a caretaker. Christopher spoke no Spanish and had never been to Mexico, but he felt guided to move to Baja. Along with his father and stepmother, they drove 1,000 miles south from San Diego to live off the desert land in the quaint but sleepy village of Todos Santos (which means "all saints").

Living close to nature was the name of the game. We lived the way we wanted to, outside. We built and rented out thatched bungalows for some income and people noticed. It became a traveler destination, yogic hostel, and eventually an informal [center for] training.

More divine intervention followed. An early guest was one of the creators of the soon-to-be-launched Yoga Alliance, the world's only yoga accrediting and certification organization. She felt the Perkinses' style of training was what the yoga world needed: a place where people could immerse themselves in the precepts of yoga philosophy and live and learn the authentic, traditional yogic practices rather than it being a teacher training factory.

The Perkinses' formal training offerings developed parallel to the establishment of the nonprofit Yoga Alliance. In 2002, Christopher and his parents launched Yandara as one of the earliest Yoga Alliance-accredited institutes in the world.

Four years later, the family bought pristine beachfront property almost fourteen miles from Todos Santos to house the growing Yandara Institute, its students, and staff.

Like an oasis, Yandara comes into view after hiking or riding up an unpaved road about a mile off the freeway. The closest hamlet is a fifteen-minute drive away, and Todos Santos is now a popular destination. There is no city for an hour in any direction.

The Perkinses' four acres are off the grid, but Christopher's older brother, Jon—who later left a successful career in Vancouver to join them—equipped the land with high-grade Wi-Fi, reliable solar power, and an uninterrupted supply of well water.

Palm trees surround the institute, along with stunning sunrises and sunsets, the scent of the ocean air, and the sounds of cowbells. Guest accommodations are comfortable glamping tents with beds and reading lights. The classroom spaces, bathrooms and kitchen are modernized thatched-roof buildings.

Christopher is the primary innovator and instructor at his home base in Mexico and satellite retreat sites in Sweden, Hawaii and Bali. Since the institute's inception, more than four thousand individuals from around the world have graduated from Yandara's primary or advanced yoga teacher training programs. Others visit for accredited workshops or retreats.

Alumni benefit from Christopher's approach to meditation, which is neither formulaic, rigid nor one-dimensional. Rather, it is more attitudinal and lifestyle-oriented and may include walking on the beach or mountain gazing.

The Guru's Wisdom: Commit to Inner Screen Time

Christopher was one of the lucky ones to whom mindfulness was part of his normal routine as a young boy. His story is proof that kids can enjoy and benefit from meditation.

> In my experience, [meditation] was not something I was ever told to do. But I was intrigued because of the loving presence of my teacher and the reality of early loss. Children are naturally closer to true meditation than many of us adult meditators may ever hope to be. I think many children would benefit from some inner screen time as well as experiencing more nature with good healthy exercise and diet.

Children are less intimidated by meditation because they are not judging themselves, comparing themselves to any ideal, or jumping to conclusions. There is no right or wrong when it comes to mindfulness.

Many adults fret they are not meditating correctly, so they dull their minds with alcohol, electronic devices, or extreme workouts. The thought of sitting in stillness like the Buddha may turn them off. As a result, few truly explore the diverse avenues of mindfulness.

Christopher uses an analogy of cleaning the house to explain pushing through beginners' angst. You don't stop and give up when the place is a complete mess. You start in one room or with a specific task, like sweeping, vacuuming or washing the laundry. Getting flustered, frozen or running away from what needs to be done only makes things worse. The same is true with mindfulness.

I first experienced Christopher's novel approach more than a decade ago. The imprint is with me daily.

In one activity, our group of teachers-in-training was blind-folded. For fifteen or twenty minutes, we walked around the beach using our invisible antennae to steer us clear of the water and prevent us from bumping into one other or stumbling over rocks. Despite our insecurities, there were no collisions or accidents. We tuned out inconsequential thoughts and tuned into the environment. Furthermore, we squelched our inner voices of doubt and fear and employed our sense of smell, sound and connection to the ground we walked on.

Another exercise took me to a clifftop overlooking the Pacific. As I sat there for half an hour, I ignored the sound, colors and energy of the ocean. The peak and I became one, and heaven was so close. I saw my deceased father, the epitome of strength and stoicism, within me. That connection to my dad made me feel as solid, secure and grounded as the mountain.

A third memorable experience was a vision quest that lasted close to twenty-four hours. Christopher led our group in a twilight send-off ceremony. He gave us each a bottle of water and a set of rules as we were led off the Yandara premises to a deserted strip of land. We were to find seclusion, stay away from each other, eat nothing, and be one with the environment.

I relished the silence and alone time of that exercise. However, my challenge was to keep warm. At night, the temperature dipped below 50°F. I had no tent, sleeping bag or gear. I wore a hat and a heavy sweater with an extra pair of socks on my hands. But that did not protect me from the biting wind. Even though I was a big city girl, I found my animal nature. I dug a trench in the sand with my hands and feet and slept burrowed like a rabbit.

As you can see, we didn't sit on a cushion or listen to a guided meditation in any of these three experiences. Instead, we received simple instructions and a gentle push to find our way.

While the above examples are not for daily practice, Christopher encourages taking meditation off the mat or cushion and into your routine. Being mindful as part of your nature will eventually make you mindful from the moment you wake until you fall asleep.

Inner freedom comes with concentration regardless of what is going on around you. Although some meditation coaches suggest people have a certain time and spot to practice each day, Christopher does not clock in. His practice is on autopilot. He may not be in a trance or with his eyes closed or in a meditative sit, but he endeavors to live a life in which he always maintains a certain level of self-awareness.

> I watch my responses to daily life so I can adjust accordingly, in real-time, to accept and release any tensions as soon as they arise, apologize if need be, and allow the flow inward to begin again. It is common for me to lose sight of a formal sitting practice, but when I do [a proper meditative sit], the extra benefit is exquisite.

Christopher notes that there can be emotional ups and downs with mindfulness practice, but the result will always be positive. Just like training for a marathon, sometimes you have muscle soreness, but the aches signify conditioning.

> Tracking emotional responses to common challenges in my daily life led me to look deeper. I investigated my motivations behind normal pursuits and the breadcrumbs took me to my inner child and a subtle yet significant lack of self-confidence. This was a tough pill to swallow at first, but

with guidance through dedicated mindfulness, breath practices, and self-inquiry, I have been able to process much of the original pain in my life.

It is helpful to establish emotional safety if there is a struggle that can be attributed to the suffering of an inner child—and too often there is. One suggestion he has for dealing with these situations is to visualize that innocent person from a distance and learn to attend to their needs intuitively.

Some of Christopher's lessons come from tantra yoga. The sacred teachings date back to 500 BC, and they are esoteric and often misunderstood. The word *tantra* means "weaving together." The practice is about delving into the spiritual and psychophysical nature of the mind to create a deeper relationship with the self.

> [Tantric traditions] pointed to the simple yet profound truth that every part of my experience can be the object of my attention. Therefore, my meditation and subsequent inner peace are not dependent on particular circumstances. This unique way of being can begin with simple mindfulness.

Human nature is not without challenges. Christopher adds:

> Acceptance includes accepting that we are humans with pain, and we are also wired to be kind, honest and helpful. We need to start small with things that are challenging yet relatively easy to accept. (For example, ending up in the slow line or missing out on the last piece of your favorite treat.) As this skill progresses, we can apply the same quality of acceptance to bigger and bigger challenges.

The master teacher has four decades of self-assessment, including twenty years of observation and validation with thousands of his students. Across the board, he finds mindfulness is a key to greater success in any endeavor when it is applied properly.

> Though I was always a fairly happy person growing up, mindfulness has revealed that my idea of happiness was just the tip of the iceberg.

We don't live in isolation. Mindfulness can improve relationships with friends, family, partners and coworkers.

> The most important result from meditation has been being able to experience what's coming up within my relationship challenges and not project my issues onto my partner or blame her for what my reactions might be. Mindfulness gives space to choose more intentionally how to communicate what I'm wanting to say. It's really where the rubber meets the road.

In other words, do yourself and those around you a favor. Bring mindfulness into your daily life.

Christopher Perkins's Five Easy Tips

1. Learn to enjoy breathing.
   Find pleasure in what most ignore. Our breath is our life force. Feel gratitude throughout your body with every inhalation and exhalation.

2. Apply deep acceptance.
   Regardless of the type of mindfulness you choose, be patient with yourself. Accept whatever arises and remember: your state of being and mind are always changing.

3. Find a place to start.
   Incorporate simple and short mindfulness
   techniques whenever and wherever you can. Practice
   without judgment.

4. Be present.
   Show up for what is going on inside and outside. If
   you begin to fret about the past or the imagined
   future, release those nagging concerns. Acknowledge
   the wandering mind and reconnect through a
   mindfulness technique that you enjoy. Life has a lot
   to offer, and we must be present to receive it.

5. Do not force it.
   Accept where you are and what feels right for you. If
   that means you need help, then so be it.

The Comforting Blanket of Meditation

My Ayurvedic constitution leans toward *vata*[5] overload
(explained further in "Chapter 6: Go with Your Gut"). I am like
the Energizer bunny, wound up at high speed until the battery
dies and I collapse. When the battery is strong, I feel invincible, even though my body is enduring a maelstrom. I have to
make an effort to nourish myself and find inner balance.

For many, stillness and quiet seem to go against the grain.
It is easier to be busy, whereas stillness is a chore and deemed
unproductive. Hot and sweaty physical yoga classes are all the
rage, while meditation is sidelined.

Most of us need gentle tugs on the parasympathetic system
to suppress the fight-or-flight response when it kicks in. Often,
in that state, the on-switch keeps getting triggered. When I
find myself in situations where the fear mode wants to take
over, I meditate and reestablish a feeling of calm. I first tapped

into the power of meditation nearly fifty years ago. This has been a lifesaver for me during oral surgery or in near-miss traffic accidents. I also rely on mindfulness techniques when I feel irritation or anger trying to surface during more common daily experiences.

For example, Susan (not her real name) acted as if she out-ranked me in the workplace, even though we were both team leaders. As ten of us prepared for a major presentation, Susan took control of the whole shebang, including the minutiae. As we were in our final dress rehearsal, awaiting the clients, she bossed us around with repeated prickly denigrations. There was no pep talk. She was belittling, rude and disrespectful, and her darts hit me too many times. Even though my modus operandi is to let that sort of thing go, my patience was at its breaking point. I wanted to wring her neck.

Instead, I took a ten-minute break. I went into my office, shut the door, and muted my phone. Then I sat cross-legged in my rolling desk chair, relaxed my eyes, and counted my inhalations and exhalations. Genuine contentedness emerged.

When I returned to the conference room, I felt lighthearted and light-footed. I floated back with an almost angelic image of Susan, wanting to give her a warm, compassionate hug.

While I no longer face a barrage of negative remarks daily, life is never devoid of stressors. However, we can choose how to respond. The body cannot heal itself when it is grappling with stress, which is why meditation is an important component of physical well-being.

In another incident in an isolated no-stoplight town in Central America, an aggressive dog pierced its big, jagged teeth into my calf. The next month, I spilled boiling water on my upper arm in the predawn hours causing a second-degree burn. While I did not ignore first aid treatments and medical care for both the bite and the burn, I turned to mantra meditation[6] for several hours daily to hasten the healing and reduce my worries.

One of the beauties of mantra meditation is it can be practiced anywhere and can be imperceptible to others. I repeated a kundalini healing mantra in bed, in the sun, wading in the ocean, and as I held a yoga pose in the sand or seated on a rock. These mindful practices also included visualization, which is known to contribute to healing. According to Johns Hopkins Medicine:

> The mind is a powerful healing tool... By creating images in your mind, you can reduce pain and other symptoms tied to your condition.[7]

When I am in the best of health, meditation is not a remedy, but my daily vitamin. My routine includes breathwork before sunrise, then *japa* (the meditative repetition of a mantra or a divine name), often combined with a nature walk. During the day, I toggle back and forth with mantra, japa and mindfulness. At night, I return to my mantras and breathwork.

There are mounds of research papers about the power of mindfulness. The impact on the brain varies depending on the type of meditation practice. Mindfulness is associated with the cortex, whose size is positively affected, as well as the patterns and degree of cortical folds. The more years of meditation practice, the more folds and patterns there are.[8]

When Christopher was a young boy, it was rare for children his age in the West to meditate. Now, many school systems encourage the practice because evidence points to its efficacy.

At one workshop I attended with Sat Bir Singh Khalsa, who you'll meet in the next chapter, he played an excerpt from a conference with the former US Surgeon General, Vivek Murthy. Dr. Murthy spoke to the director of the National Institutes of Health about the merits of Eastern practices.[9] Dr. Murthy referred to cases where meditation made significant differences in schoolchildren.

In the excerpt, the surgeon general shared how he had visited a public school surrounded by crime. Violence took the lives of fifty people near the campus in just one year. When the killers started dumping dead bodies on the school grounds, the administration became desperate. While the schools could not stop the gang warfare, they found they could protect the kids' emotions and assuage their grief with meditation.

The effect was a marked reduction in violence and an increase in students' performance. The principal noted improvement within just two weeks. Over one year, the suspension rate dropped in half. Parents were surprised their children were not lashing out like they used to. The kids recognized the benefits too. As a result, 95 percent of them signed up again for meditation the next term.

From schools to businesses, meditation makes a difference. A 2020 article in *Forbes* magazine named multiple reasons meditation is beneficial in the workplace.[10] The author, Laura Sage, cites a University of California, Davis, study that recognized meditation contributed to reduced stress and cortisol levels and increased cognition.[11] Group practices increased collaboration, innovation and quality of work. Mindfulness can boost memory and curb emotional reactions. The research also showed the practice has a positive effect on prosocial behaviors, leading to reduced prejudice—all elements that our world sorely needs.

||||||||||||||||||||||||||||||||||||||||||||||||||||||||||||||||||||||||||||||||||||||||||||||||||||||||||||||||||||||||||||||||||||||

Give It a Try:
Take a One-Minute Time-Out

Mindfulness can be practiced almost anywhere, anytime. The following simple exercises are intended to be repeated multiple times a day, for as little as a minute at a time. Give them all a fair chance to see which fits your temperament and lifestyle best. If you seem to get off track, simply start again with renewed enthusiasm. There is no right or wrong way. As you get comfortable with one or more of these mindfulness techniques, extend the time you practice them.

Once you have found your favorite and take some time learning how it works best for you, you have a new life hack. Whenever the slightest bit of tension or stress arises, use this tool to nip it in the bud. It may be good to schedule one-minute minibreaks throughout the day to practice. Better yet, download a mindfulness app to remind you. When the alert sounds, whatever you are doing, take a sixty-second time-out.

For those who are forever attached to their devices, Christopher suggests a one-minute mindfulness practice each time you reach for your phone or before you log on to your computer. Here are some options to chose from.

- **Count one, two, three.**
  Track just three conscious breaths in a row with single-pointed awareness. Start with any one breath at any time. It could be the breath you are breathing in now. Let it flow in and flow out naturally. Just concentrate for three inhalations and you are done.

- **Disconnect from everything but the breath.**
  Take in a very slow, deep breath. Release any thoughts or feelings that surface, other than the sensation of

the oxygen entering and leaving your body. Should any extraneous thoughts arise, accept them, and redirect your focus to the air entering and exiting your nose. Endeavor to engage with the breath and nothing else.

- **Label the movement of oxygen.**
  Silently repeat, "I am inhaling, I am exhaling." Or count each breath. "Inhale one, exhale one. Inhale two, exhale two." When you get to ten, return to one, rather than going on to eleven.

- **Follow your breath.**
  Pay attention to the sensation of cool air entering your nose or mouth. Feel the breath descend the throat and throughout the body. Imagine the palms of your hands, the soles of your feet, or the crown of your head soaking up all the energy from the universe (also known as "prana" or "qi") with each inhalation. When you exhale, visualize the breath cleansing every cell of your body.

- **Visualize peace within.**
  Connect to elements of nature that resonate with you, regardless of if you are sitting in an office cubicle or weeding in your backyard. Draw a picture in your mind and see yourself within the frame for at least a minute. Be still like a tree. Flow like a river. Focus like an eagle. Be soft like a cat or brave like a lion.

- **Synchronize simple body movements with breath.**
  Seated or standing, with each inhalation, lengthen the spine and arch the back. As you exhale, relax and allow the chin to hang toward the chest, rounding

the back. Or, with each breath in, reach your hands up to the sky, and with each exhalation roll down, bend the knees, and let the fingertips touch the floor. Don't rush. Relish each breath. Repeat for five or six rounds.

- **Breathe in and out, with just one nostril.**
  Two common alternate nostril breathing techniques[12] are *anuloma viloma* (with and against the flow) and *nadi shodana* (channel cleaning). There are different ways to practice these two forms of pranayama, but they each focus on the inhalation and exhalation through one nostril at a time. The simplest way is to hold your right hand in front of your face, palm toward your nose. Alternate pinching your right nostril shut with your thumb while inhaling fully through the left nostril, then closing your left nostril with your pinky and ring finger while exhaling through the right side. For the next round, begin by inhaling through the right, and exhaling through the left. Try ten rounds to start.

- **Repeat, repeat, repeat.**
  Japa is the repetition of a few sacred words or a mantra. Sometimes, a master prescribes the mantra to a student. A simple peace mantra that many yoga classes end with is "Om[13] shanti[14] shanti shanti om." Count each utterance of the mantra by pushing one bead on your strand of 108 mala beads. Each round equals 108 repetitions, which is considered an auspicious number. Japa is often practiced in a near whisper throughout the day, with or without the beads. One round, depending on your speed, takes

three or four minutes. If you use a rosary with fifty-four beads, it should need less than two minutes.

- **Label the activity of the senses.**
  As you sit in silence, lie down or walk, pay attention to all your senses one by one. Listen. See. Feel. Taste. Smell. Choose times throughout the day to integrate this gentle awareness into your routine.

- **Scan your physical body.**
  Start at your head and concentrate for a moment on how it feels. Slowly, work your way down. Without moving, relax each part of your body through the neck, shoulders, upper arms, torso and legs. When you reach your toes, reverse direction and go back up to the crown of your head. It may help to name your body parts and organs silently.

Whichever techniques you choose, remember, there is no destination. Enjoy the journey. Unwind and experience more of this precious human life, day by day, minute by minute.

Without a doubt, the mind can act as your best friend or worst enemy. You have the power to use it to your advantage. In fact, as you're about to see, you can rewire your brain.

Chapter 2: Yoga as an Emotional Lifesaver

Yoga is providing benefits that
most of modern medicine does not.

—Dr. Sat Bir Singh Khalsa

The life mission of Sat Bir Singh Khalsa, PhD, has been to corroborate the efficacy of yoga. He is the director of research for Yoga Alliance and also a Harvard Medical School associate professor. As a neuroscientist, he is relentless in digging for scientific evidence to prove the wisdom of the sages. Affiliated with the greatest names in medicine and integrative health, he dissects different aspects of the ancient technique of yoga—in particular, its interactions with the brain. He is an encyclopedia of academic work and clinical studies and a principal investigator in milestone yogic research.

Depression, post-traumatic stress disorder (PTSD) and anxiety are among the most common mental or behavioral health issues. Dr. Khalsa has spent years amassing evidence for why yoga is one of the best approaches to manage these conditions. His studies show that yoga delivers enhanced clarity and buoyed emotional well-being, making the ancient practice sometimes more effective than modern treatments.

One of my greatest sources of professional development is the International Association of Yoga Therapists' multiday Symposium on Yoga Therapy and Research conferences.

Dr. Khalsa, editor-in-chief of the organization's *International Journal of Yoga Therapy*, was a plenary speaker at the conference in 2015 and 2017 in Newport Beach, California. Aware of his reputation, I made a beeline for the researcher's lectures. The first year, he also led a session on kundalini yoga for anxiety. Thanks to my copious note-taking habit, I later coached clients with severe PTSD in breath and bodywork exercises I picked up from that one class with Dr. Khalsa.

When the neuroscientist took part in San Antonio's first International Day of Yoga in 2017, I volunteered to promote his seminar for physicians, students and healthcare professionals. A year later, I later jumped at the opportunity to attend an entire weekend of presentations and therapeutic kundalini-based practices with Dr. Khalsa in Austin, Texas. Over the following years, he offered dozens of virtual sessions, and I signed up for them all.

I'm a reader and writer, not a numbers person. Seeing slide after slide of bar graphs, pie charts, line charts, histograms and raw statistics is not my favorite way to learn. Despite Dr. Khalsa's data-driven content, every hour hearing him taught me invaluable knowledge. The tall, slim research guru dressed in all-white loose clothing and turban with his never-cut hair and beard can explain decades of research studies and personalize the evidence and outcomes, leaving you asking, "Why on earth doesn't the whole world know about this?"

He is the quintessential pragmatic scientist, and yet he lives and breathes in a spiritual world. His career brings these two realities into one. I know of no other person who has dug so deep into the data to prove the innumerable benefits of yoga. But his focus is not on its impact on the muscles, connective tissues, circulatory system, or bones. His focus is on the brain.

The Inquisitive Yogi: Dr. Sat Bir Singh Khalsa

A much younger Khalsa was intrigued by the connection between yoga and the brain long before the Eastern practice became popular in every gym.

He grew up in Canada in the '60s. It was the psychedelic era of tie-dyed apparel, Peter Max pop art, magic mushrooms, illegal marijuana, and the rock music of Jefferson Airplane, Jimi Hendrix and Janis Joplin. Thinking outside of the box and living beyond the white picket fence were growing in popularity among the younger generation. Youth were breaking away from traditional roles, rules and expectations. There was a disconnect between the real world and the lifestyles flaunted on the television screens. Hippies and yippies had little in common with Mayberry Sheriff Andy Taylor, single dad to Opie (played by a very young Ron Howard). Nor did young women aspire to a life like June Cleaver, the mom from *Leave It to Beaver*, decked out in pearls, a dress and high heels as she prepared the family dinner.

Dr. Khalsa recalls:

> I was living in the counterculture. I wasn't alone at this point in time. When I was in high school, I was a "long hair," thinking there's got to be more than a three-car garage in my future. There's got to be more depth and meaning in life.

Eastern philosophy and practices floated over to the West. During the time of flower-power and Beatlemania, the Fab Four went to India to immerse themselves in yoga and transcendental meditation. The idols from Liverpool incorporated Sanskrit verses to songs like "Across the Universe" and "My Sweet Lord." "Norwegian Wood" was the first of the rock stars' music to feature the sounds of the sitar.[15] Indian spirituality influenced their attire, album covers, and even belief systems. In reality, Indian gurus and swamis had already sensed the need for something different among Westerners. The youth movement stateside was ready for alternative ways of thinking about themselves and humanity.

Philip Goldberg, author of *American Veda*,[16] attests the Beatles revolution stretched far beyond the record players.

> Overnight, everyone knew what the word "mantra" meant. People now knew there was something called meditation. Within five years, meditation was no longer a counterculture hippie thing. The demand for these teachings grew overnight—and exponentially—after the Beatles.

> When the Beatles went to India, there were only twelve people who could teach transcendental meditation [in the United States]. Then, there were thousands—like me. The disenfranchised younger generation said to themselves, "If the Beatles can go off and spend time in Rishikesh, [India,] then there must be something to this."

That was the scenario as the young Canadian kept searching and doing his homework. He took a college course in the philosophy of mysticism, which led him to immerse himself in books about human consciousness and the cross section of religion, spirituality and human behavior.

Khalsa was intrigued by the legendary psychologist William James, author of *The Varieties of Religious Experience*; Abraham Maslow, who penned *Religions, Values, and Peak Experiences*; and Alan Watts's *The Way of Zen.* Turned off by what many deemed to be dogma and ritual, he developed a newfound respect for the deeper contemplative experiences that were originally the goal of religions.

I understood more of what religion and spirituality were about. At one point, I said it was time to stop reading and start doing. Reading is inspiring, but it won't give you that contemplative experience.

When the University of Toronto science major found yoga among the course offerings, he registered without hesitation. Earning college credit hours for yoga was like "a message from the sky" for the co-ed. Just a few years later, at twenty-three, he began teaching *kundalini* yoga, an energetic practice that integrates breathwork with mantra meditation and movement.

Absorbed in the practice and lifestyle of a yogi, learning philosophy and attending yoga classes and workshops, young Khalsa moved into an *ashram*, a center for spiritual study, where he could fully engage. After a few years, his inclination led him to return to his passion for science. His goal? Uncover the mysteries behind the ancient yogic teachings. He was met with isolation and occasional external resistance, as the benefits of yoga were of minimal interest to most people.

Undeterred, he continued his post-grad studies in conventional physiology and neuroscience, as he put his curiosity about the intersection of yoga and altered states on the shelf for the short term.

By 1985, the year Khalsa earned his PhD, Dr. Herbert Benson, a Harvard Medical School professor, penned two best-sellers on the relaxation response. Khalsa aspired to learn from the mind/body medicine pioneer whose seminal investigations he admired. However, Dr. Benson was not taking on any students who were not medical doctors, so Khalsa headed to the University of Virginia to pursue postdoctoral studies on biological rhythms and sleep. He worked east of the Blue Ridge Mountains for the next ten years, helping to build the university's importance as a brain and neuroscience research facility.

In 1996, he transitioned to a lab at Harvard Medical School and the puzzle pieces started falling into place. Five years later, the National Center for Complementary and Alternative Health, a division of the National Institutes of Health (NIH), finally began funding yoga research and awarded him a five-year grant to study the connection between yoga and sleep disorders. That was the first of several grants he would receive from NIH to explore yoga and the brain.

And years later, Dr. Khalsa finally collaborated with the esteemed Dr. Benson on both a research grant and a mind/body medicine course.

The Guru's Wisdom: Rewire the Brain

Westerners don't always know what they are getting into when they take their first yoga class. Too often, people don't recognize the scale and scope of the practice. Most Americans equate yoga with physical exercise. But the true meaning of the word *yoga* is "union." The authentic philosophical and holistic approach links the mind, body and spirit—and so much more.

Dr. Khalsa says it is common for people to give yoga a shot for specific physical reasons to improve their health and well-being. Maybe it's to heal a tennis elbow, an injured knee, a nagging backache, or to lose a few extra inches around the tummy or hips. Although yoga can address those physical concerns, the practice often generates a surprise payoff—its powerful impact on mental well-being.

The image of the happy Buddha or a Zen-like monk sitting in a state of calm amid chaos is not just a stereotype. In a national survey of yoga practitioners, almost 90 percent said they are happier because they remain involved in the ancient tradition.

To those that stay with the practice, it is not uncommon to emerge from a funk and experience enhanced self-regulation, stress resilience, mind/body awareness, well-being and other positive psychological states. Dr. Khalsa says those positive results are based on changes in the central nervous system, biochemistry and brain structure. Yoga literally changes the brain.

While there are many branches and tenets to the ancient art, when Dr. Khalsa refers to yoga, he views it in terms of:

- postures/exercise
- breathwork
- relaxation
- meditation

Not one facet or another, but all four in unison.

This time-honored brain tonic is neither fancy nor expensive. As yoga was handed down from the masters, there is no need for special gear, props or settings—just intent, commitment and regularity of practice.

Subduing the Symptoms of Post-Traumatic Stress Disorder

PTSD is not a new condition; it just changed names. The WWI generation called the disorder "shell shock." WWII era referred to PTSD by the misnomers of "combat stress reaction," "soldier's heart," "battle fatigue," "combat neurosis," and "war neuroses." Now we understand PTSD is not just a military man's illness. The mental health condition cuts across gender, ethnicity, geographical, professional and socioeconomic groups. Chances are, you or someone you know has experienced this disorder.

PTSD is a chronic condition that stems from traumatic emotional or physical shocks, pains or injuries. In the United States, 60 percent of males and 50 percent of females face trauma in their lives.[17] While the types of trauma vary, PTSD presents in 8 percent of American women versus 4 percent of men. That correlates to thirteen million adults from all walks of life engaging in a battle with this mental health condition each year in America.[18]

Dr. Khalsa explains that:

> Trauma occurs when somebody experiences a life-threatening event. It can be a single event or a series of events. There's a gradation of levels of trauma. It can be short-term post-traumatic stress or a bona fide clinical disorder. There are both physical and mental cognitive effects [especially as] people reexperience the trauma in flashbacks by day or nightmares at night.

There is a wide range of circumstances that contribute to PTSD. For some, the cause is repeated, adverse plights from childhood, like sexual abuse or molestation. Other times, the misfortunes arise as an adult. Being a victim of or witnessing violence can precipitate the condition. That's why the injury—and trauma *is* classified as an injury—haunts hospital emergency room employees and first responders.

Just as our fingerprints are different, so are our reactions. The repercussions for two soldiers in an ambush, or thousands witnessing the fall of the Twin Towers in Manhattan on 9/11, are not alike. That is because of a resiliency factor, the ability to process, react and move beyond the shock or aggression without permanent injury.

Everyone has different response mechanisms. When the range of what someone can tolerate is exceeded, they can develop PTSD. For example, children with high exposure to unresolved traumatic events may experience dysregulated emotional responses that can be expressed as an outpouring of frustration, sadness, aggression or anger. That inability to control one's emotions can be lifelong.

There's a host of psychological and physical symptoms associated with PTSD. The disorder can affect the body with disruptive panic attacks, nausea, violent outbursts, hyperarousal, dizziness, a racing heart, or chronic pain. Meanwhile, the emotional responses can be harder to decipher. Those can range from feelings of detachment, guilt or shame to emotional numbness or poor concentration.

According to Dr. Khalsa, conventional treatments are one-sided and often ineffective. In fact, antidepressants only work 42 percent of the time for those with the disorder.

Many people dealing with PTSD find exercise helpful, but yoga's benefits outdeliver those of traditional physical workouts. The scores of different yoga styles and flavors of the day can be confusing. The menu board on a yoga studio schedule may include a dozen different names of classes, many of which are in Sanskrit, like hatha, yoga nidra, tantra, ananda, Anusara, Jivamukti, Iyengar, kundalini, ashtanga, vinyasa and viniyoga.

Many of the more modern styles of yoga omit the breathwork or meditation, or downplay the importance of relaxation.

Dr. Khalsa says that concentrating on all four components of yoga (postures, breathing, relaxation and meditation) has psychological and physical benefits that counteract traumatic stress disorder and trauma. While each component of yoga has its benefits, when the four are performed in unison, the positive impact is greater.

Movement and relaxation can release physical and emotional tensions. Slow mindful yogic breathing affects the autonomic system and soothes hyperarousal. Furthermore, meditation leads to metacognition (the awareness of one's thought processes) and inspires positive psychological, physiological and spiritual effects.

> Meditation, by definition, is the relaxed nonanalytical focus of attention. Regardless of the style, if you are practicing meditation properly, you are letting your thoughts go. With practice over time, you acquire more self-regulation of your thoughts and emotions and ultimately achieve a state of metacognition, or the understanding or experience that you are more than your thoughts. That's what cognitive behavioral therapy (CBT)[19] is all about: understanding that your thoughts are just thoughts.

Yoga normalizes human cognitive function in a nonthreatening manner, whereas traditional mental health therapies often directly confront the fear, memory or trigger with reexposure to the trauma. For those with PTSD, talking about or reliving the incident can be retraumatizing and distressing.

Most certified yoga therapists and trauma-informed instructors are sensitive to potential triggers. Plus, yoga is designed not to provoke the rehashing that can spark flare-ups.

> The work is done behind the curtain. You do the yoga for eight weeks and your PTSD symptoms have improved. You don't know what happened, but you're no longer having flashbacks and you're no longer hyperaroused.

In one of Dr. Khalsa's randomized control trials, perceived stress diminished while resiliency, a major factor in how PTSD manifests, improved.[20] There was also a notable overall drop in common related symptoms, including depression, anxiety and stress. Furthermore, Khalsa notes that a study among military personnel indicated the holistic yoga approach lessened unhealthy avoidance symptoms, hyperarousal, flashbacks and nightmares while slightly improving resiliency, positivity and mindfulness.[21]

One US Army Desert Storm veteran from Dr. Khalsa's trials said yoga improved his temper.

> I loved it. I felt full of energy and didn't feel stressed out. I felt very motivated. It brought down my stress level. I was more focused and more understanding.

Meanwhile, on the other side of the globe, yoga researchers assessed PTSD among 183 tsunami survivors.[22] After just one week of yogic breathing, investigators noted improvements in their condition. Six weeks later, the participants' symptoms were under control, whereas those not doing the breathwork showed no improvement in PTSD indicators.

These are just a sampling of studies that attest to the power of yoga in treating this disorder. Research bears witness that yoga improves self-regulation, mind/body awareness, resiliency and serenity, all of which are key ingredients in managing PTSD.

From Feeling Blue to Feeling Blissful

Worldwide, two hundred eighty million people suffer from depression.[23] The often stress-related condition affects about twice as many females in the fourteen to twenty-five age bracket as males, but these prevalence rates decrease with age.[24] Yet that number will increase with pregnancy when 70 to 80 percent of women will experience the baby blues,[25] and one in seven will battle major depression after childbirth, according to the American Pregnancy Association.[26]

Gloominess is not always clinical depression, Dr. Khalsa explains.

> Depression refers to a depressed mood. Often people will describe this as feeling down or blue. It's a very common experience in everyday life and often associated with life events.
>
> Depression becomes clinically significant when it interferes regularly with daily activities related to work, family, recreation, sleep, levels of attention, appetite, energy or cognitive activity, as well as increasing feelings of guilt or remorse or physical agitation.

The depths of depression worsen with rumination, the nagging images, thoughts or fears that keep replaying in your head. Rumination is like a hamster on a wheel; you're unable to escape it. The nonstop negative churning can provoke anxiety and then depression if it's not interrupted or replaced with positive thought patterns.

Reducing or erasing ruminations and gloomy mental images rekindles emotional stability.

> One of the most powerful forms of psychotherapy for depression is cognitive behavioral therapy, which addresses the specific thought processes inherent in the disorder. Yoga's meditative component allows for the development of self-regulation of thought processes. That's a shared principle between CBT and yoga. Ultimately, these practices lead to metacognition and the ability to be aware of and regulate your thought processes more effectively.

As we saw with PTSD, medications aren't always the answer.[27] Dr. Khalsa warns:

> There's a subpopulation of people with depression who have a certain genetic makeup that makes them more resistant to treatment by pharmaceuticals. So yoga has a [role] to play here.

Blissfulness is in the brain. Physical movement, as done in a hatha class,[28] and yogic breathing techniques each contribute to regulating the amygdala, a region in the brain's temporal lobe that can stir up emotions. When it comes to the amygdala, bigger is not better. An overactive amygdala correlates to depression and post-traumatic stress flare-ups. Yoga shrinks this almond-shaped mass of gray matter, preventing reactions from blowing up.

What's more, this practice that dates back thousands of years regulates the brain's chemical messengers. Several studies corroborate how yoga turns on the gamma-aminobutyric acid (GABA) neurotransmitter that blocks nervous system activity. Increased GABA produces a state of calm. Decreased GABA can lead to depression, anxiety and sleep disorders.

Just one hour of yoga can make a difference. A Boston University School of Medicine researcher found that a single Iyengar yoga class[29] can boost the levels of brain GABA. Those suffering from major depressive disorder showed improved GABA levels that lasted for eight days after each yoga session.[30]

One reason many attend a yoga and meditation retreat is to relish that sense of immense calm. The heavenly feeling is not just about escaping the daily home and work routine. Something wonderful happens to your brain when you practice yoga.

A report in *Frontiers in Human Neuroscience* explored the positive impact of meditative retreats.[31] There were measurable changes in the cortisol levels and neuroplasticity of retreat attendees. It is believed that when the brain lacks neuroplasticity (that ability to remodel, reorganize and rewire itself), mental illnesses arise, including depression and anxiety.

Yoga leads to heightened levels of self-awareness and concentration. According to Dr. Khalsa:

> A continuously wandering mind is an unhappy mind because of the persistent negative content of many of our thoughts. The more you are able to self-regulate thought processes, the less you become emotionally and stress reactive to your thoughts. Over time, your emotional brain may actually shrink in volume due to this decreased reactivity.

Neuropsychologist and meditation teacher Rick Hanson, PhD, coined the term "hardwiring happiness" to explain how people can pull themselves out of the muck and experience inner peace, confidence and joy. In a Marin County TEDx Talk called "Hardwiring Happiness," he said, "The mind can change the brain to change the mind," which heals emotional pains and helps you enjoy life more.

Scans confirm that meditation leads to positive changes in the amygdala—which Hanson calls "the alarm bell of your brain"—and other regions of the brain, as well as increasing cerebral flow.[32] The core function of the autonomic nervous system (responsible for the fight-or-flight response) changes with meditation, and the duration of the practice of yoga is directly related to the structural reshaping of the brain.

Moreover, some of the effects are long-lasting and even intergenerational as the practice rewires not only the brain but our genes.

> Meditation turns on genes that are good for us. It's happening at the very core of our selves. We are changing our brains and our bodies when we meditate.

If you or someone you care about needs to get out of a rut, yoga and meditation are easy and enjoyable and can be practiced in group settings, online or by yourself. Plus, finding time for your emotional boost should not be hard to incorporate into daily life. Dr. Khalsa suggests practicing quick pick-me-ups anytime, anywhere, like doing breathwork on a bus, progressive relaxation in an elevator, or mindfulness as you go about your chores.

Yoga is transformative. During his years of practice and research, Dr. Khalsa has heard from many people that yoga not only changed their lives, it saved them. The holistic practice brings about better focus, clarity, peace and resilience. Dr. Khalsa finds, with regular practice over time, yoga practitioners become less attracted to material goals of wealth, power and fame.

These kinds of deeper changes in positive psychology, including life meaning and purpose, can [ultimately] lead to less crime, war and poverty, and that to me is the biggest potential of these practices. Modern medicine is incapable of doing this.

Dr. Khalsa's Five Easy Tips

1. **Prioritize your well-being.**
   Carve out time each day for yourself, which includes finding and tapping into as many resources as possible. Of course, if you have a diagnosed disorder, behavioral techniques in psychotherapy, such as cognitive behavioral therapy, should not be ignored.

2. **Find a meditative practice that you enjoy.**
   You don't have to be sitting cross-legged for long periods of time to meditate. Mantra meditation, walking meditation, and different mindfulness techniques are all excellent options. Several of the more traditional styles of yoga, including Sivananda, Integral, and kundalini, incorporate meditation. For beginners, the simplest way to meditate is by concentrating on each inhalation and exhalation.

3. **Incorporate breathing techniques that regulate and slow down the breath.**
   There are many styles of breathwork. Some are contraindicated for pregnant women or those with uncontrolled high blood pressure. Traditional yogic three-part breathing (described in "Give It a Try: Three-Minute Breathwork Exercise" on page 40) is generally appropriate for everyone.

4. **Pay attention to the postures.**
Yoga poses are best held with slow, deep breathing as you focus on sensations throughout your body, your breath, and minute changes in your mood. Don't judge yourself against an image in a book or online or against what your teacher or anyone else does. If you are comfortable closing your eyes, turning off the visual senses increases the ability to focus within.

5. **Enjoy relaxation.**
Undoubtedly, we all need time to shut out the world and let the body and mind restore and recalibrate. *Savasana* (corpse pose), lying flat on your back with your eyes closed, is the favorite of many. While some are uncomfortable in stillness, quieting oneself is essential for well-being, which is why all yoga classes end with up to ten minutes of relaxing savasana.

Rising from the Funk

As a yoga therapist, I don't separate the mind from the body. For my students and clients dealing with serious physical conditions, I pay even greater attention to their emotions and spirit. For example, when I work with cancer patients and survivors, I incorporate laughter yoga, yoga nidra (a.k.a. iRest),[33] socialization exercises, and gratitude practices. Above all, I try to tailor my sessions recognizing no two people are identical and people's needs and preferences shift from one day (or minute) to another.

For those awaiting lab or biopsy results, or undergoing chemotherapy or radiation, each day brings a different level of energy, emotions and comfort or discomfort. When you have the flu, you naturally want to sip hot liquids, bundle up in bed or on a couch, and withdraw rather than go skiing, partying or eating a heavy meal. Our bodies seem to tell us what they need. But it takes more effort to recognize what the mind and soul need. Our intuition works best when the body and mind are quiet, which may be why I embrace silence.

At one of those dips in a life zigzag, I wanted a pick-me-up. I found sahaja yoga when I most needed it. *Sahaja* is a simple and short standardized style of guided, or self-guided, meditation that incorporates positive affirmations. After a few years, I felt I had integrated the affirmations into my life. I tapered off my practice, but my respect for sahaja as a powerful emotional support technique remains.

Researchers from the University of Sydney conducted a meta-analysis of 910 participants and found sahaja yoga led to a significant decrease in anxiety and had a positive impact on well-being among healthy adults. The study also concluded that sahaja meditators enjoyed better overall physical and mental health, emotional and social functioning, and vitality.

Sahaja is one of countless ways to bring about a positive mental state of mind in as little as ten minutes, once or twice a day. As with anything, success is reliant on taking the first step and keeping it up.

Give It a Try:
Three-Minute Breathwork Exercise

There are a wide variety of pranayama breathing techniques, but the following is the standard yogic breath, also called "three-part breathing" or "long deep breathing." The Sanskrit name is *ujjayi*, meaning "victorious."

I try to incorporate ujjayi breath throughout my physical yoga practice. Breathwork is also my sleep tonic. If I wake up in the middle of the night or if my mind is too active at bedtime, I put my hands on my belly and zoom in on my yogic breathing. It doesn't take long before I am in dreamland.

The beauty of breathing exercises is they can be done anywhere, in any position. You can focus on the following technique in the grocery store, in an airplane, or even in the dentist's chair—whenever and wherever you need to relax.

1. **Make yourself comfortable.** If appropriate, lie down on your back to provide more space for the diaphragm to descend and retract. If seated, keep your back erect and your head in alignment with the spine.

2. **Close your eyes if it feels right for you.** Without clenching your teeth, close your mouth and relax your tongue and jaw. Then, breathe in and out through the nose.

3. **Place one palm on your lower belly and the other on your heart.** Visualize your torso as a pitcher. With each inhalation, the vessel fills from the bottom with water. Conversely, with each exhalation, the liquid pours out from the top. In other words, deflate the chest, then the upper abdomen, followed by the lower belly as you exhale. Focus on filling the body with as much fresh oxygen as possible, and then squeezing out every bit of air. Notice how the air feels entering and leaving your nostrils with each breath. Continue for several minutes. The slower your breathing, the better.

||||||||||||||||||||||||||||||||||||||||||||||||||||||||||||||||||||||||||||||||||||||||||||||||||||||||||||||||||||||||||||||||||

Give It a Try:
Relax Your Muscles

For those with anxiety, at times, the body is so tense it can be difficult to loosen up and practice breathwork. The following exercise helps to relax central muscles in the body while releasing mental tension as well.

There are multiple methods of performing progressive relaxation. I often guide my students and clients in the following manner.

1. **Lie down on your back on a mat, a rug or on your bed.**
   If you prefer, place a pillow, cushion or rolled-up blanket under your knees or head and neck.

2. **Open your eyes wide, as if in shock.**
   Hold for a few breaths, then release and feel your eyelids gently close.

3. **Open your mouth as if you are shouting.**
   Stretch your mouth and jaw as much as possible for a few breaths. Then, release without closing your jaw completely. Allow your tongue to float in your mouth and keep your jaw relaxed.

4. **Make a fist with your right hand.**
   Raise your fist off the ground a few inches. Squeeze as tightly as you can for several breaths. Imagine you are pressing every drop out of a lime held in the palm of your hand. After repeated inhalations and exhalations, relax all your fingers and allow your hand to sink to the floor. Repeat with the left hand.

5. **Squeeze your right thigh muscles as tightly as you can.**
   Feel your gluteal muscles harden and the entire right leg stiffen. Release all tension as you take a few

slow breaths. Then, let the right leg sink like a heavy anchor. Proceed on the other side.

6. **Engage your glutes on both sides.**
Imagine that they are made of steel. With every breath, try to make those muscles harder. Then, with a slow exhalation, let every inch of your body relax and melt into the ground.

7. **The final component addresses that region of our body that often harbors tension, the upper back and neck.**
Visualize a pencil between your shoulder blades. Try to hold the imaginary pencil in place by pulling the shoulder blades back and together. Your sternum should open as the upper back is engaged. Press that thin pencil as tightly as possible for multiple breaths, then gradually release and feel your entire body, head to toe, at ease. Enjoy this state of total relaxation for another minute or two, maintaining slow, deep breaths.

You've probably heard the adage "laughter is the best medicine." Now find out how one man used laughter to triumph over severe trauma, depression and chronic pain.

Chapter 3: The Magic of Laughter as Medicine

Through laughter, humans fall in love with life.[34]

—Lenín Moreno Garcés,
former Constitutional President of the
Republic of Ecuador

W hen my daughter was a baby, her father and I owned a Spanish tapas bar in Quito, Ecuador. He kept his day job. During operating hours, I managed the bare-bones kitchen and waitstaff, waited tables, bartended, manned the cash register, and befriended my customer base. At home, I maintained the ledgers and prepared desserts for the restaurant.

Two men swung by the café daily. They were business associates who rented office space above our café. One was a Midwesterner married to an Ecuadorian. The other was born in a remote Amazonian hamlet but was raised in the capital. Together, they coordinated and managed a cultural and educational exchange program. To my recollection, they recruited, prepared and coordinated visits from students in the United

States to Ecuador, and for Ecuadorian students to study in the States.

Lenín Moreno was the Ecuadorian half of the business partnership. Both men took their midday coffees, often with my homemade cheesecake topped with chocolate, at the small four-seater counter that was my primary workstation.

In 1990, we sold the business and moved to Miami. My only mementos of the café are protected in a single magnetized plastic photo album sleeve. One side showcases my sample promotional letter on our red, yellow and black letterhead. On the other side is coverage from two newspaper society editors that attended our grand opening. Each features a celebratory shot of my husband, my father-in-law and me. Although my father snapped a few black-and-white photos during one visit, those are filed among the thousands I scanned and saved on a single CD. Fortunately, almost all my memories are still vivid in my brain.

I knew Lenín Moreno long before a life of politics was on his mind. I have not seen him for thirty years, but I have avidly followed his redirection in life.

The Good-Humored President: Lenín Moreno

Around 2006, I heard that a man named Lenín Moreno was running for vice president of the Republic of Ecuador as Rafael Correa's running mate. Despite the unusual first name, I clicked on the photos and videos to be sure it was the same Lenín from my bistro. There was no doubt. After fifteen years of not being in touch, I recognized his strong *serrano* (highland) accent. His face hadn't changed except for a few more gray hairs and laugh lines. But he was confined to a wheelchair. The Lenín I knew walked up and down the flights of stairs to his office multiple times a day.

When I saw him seated in the wheelchair, I read the details from the Ecuadorian news reports. In 1998, two armed men assaulted him. One pulled the trigger, and a bullet lodged in his spine. Multiple surgeries did not alleviate his severe pain or prevent him from being primarily bedridden for almost four years. Paralyzed for life from the waist down, his doctors labeled him 100 percent disabled.

From one day to the next, his life changed. Instead of wallowing in pity and lying around depressed (which he did do at first), the paralyzed man found rehabilitation through *risoterapia* (laughter therapy). Fueled by humor, he not only pulled himself up from the depths of personal tragedy, but transformed the lives of others. In a country with no unemployment or disability benefits, Lenín was inspired by his harrowing and frustrating experiences to convert Ecuador into a role model for its work with the disabled.

After his injury, Lenín established a foundation to promote humor and positive mental attitudes, particularly among Ecuador's marginalized groups, including abandoned children, children with HIV, and food-insecure seniors. Fueled by a desire to help others, he gave motivational speeches to private and public groups. Lenín would say his disabilities gave him the strength to rise to the top.

He amassed a personal library of 1,300 titles (which later grew to 8,000) and penned and published ten of his own. Many of the books he wrote focus on humor, including *Teoría y Práctica del Humor* (*Theory and Practice of Humor*), *Ser Feliz es Fácil y Divertido* (*To Be Happy is Easy and Fun*), *Los Mejores Chistes del Mundo* (*The World's Best Jokes*), *Humor de los Famosos* (*Humor from Famous People*), and *Ríase, No Sea Enfermo* (*Laugh, Don't be Sick*).

In January 2007, he took office as vice president of the Republic of Ecuador under Rafael Correa. In 2013, Vice President Moreno resigned and moved to Geneva, Switzerland, when United Nations Secretary-General Ban Ki-Moon appointed him Special Envoy on Disability and Accessibility. His commitment to improving the world for the differently abled population was not ignored. He received multiple advanced honorary degrees and was a Nobel Peace Prize nominee.

In 2016, Moreno was encouraged by many to return to Carondelet (the Ecuadorian equivalent of the US White House). He jokes people said "the table was set," meaning it would be an easy victory for the presidency. His response, "There wasn't even a table," made it clear that he had a long road ahead of him. However, confident he could make a positive impact on his homeland, he left Geneva, won the elections, and served as Constitutional President of the Republic of Ecuador from 2017 to 2021. On his inauguration day, he became the first Latin American paraplegic president and the only living head of state confined to a wheelchair.

Politics can be a messy business in any country. Although Lenín didn't escape the political fire after he left office, I do not judge him for his role as an elected official. Rather, I have incredible respect for how he overcame exceptional challenges in his life and never stopped advocating for others.

Throughout his tenure as an elected official, he not only worked to improve the lives of the disabled but also to uplift the emotional well-being of the average Ecuadorian. When he ran for the presidency, his proposed plans could have been from a spiritual self-help book. He spoke of the need for citizens to have pride and joy, healthy and happy families, and to honor and respect the beauty in diversity.

His platform was about consensus building and kindness. His slogan, "*Toda Una Vida*," meaning "an entire lifetime," was taken from a classic Los Panchos hit from the 1940s, rerecorded by Mexican pop idol Luis Miguel in 2001. Under President Moreno, that popular song title referred to caring for citizens from conception until their final breaths.

The branding of President Moreno's campaign objectives shouted warmth and positivity. For example, "*Misión Ternura*" ("Mission of Tenderness") was the catchy name of his prenatal, neonatal and early childhood plan. In his inaugural address, he assured the public:

> From their first steps, we will instill values and foster a love for science, knowledge, technology and sport. Not just body-building, but a road to strengthening one's will... a passion that gives them a sense of self-worth so they don't need to reach out for unseemly substances.

He created similar platforms for other age groups. He billed the adolescent campaign "*Impulso Joven*" ("The Momentum of Youth") and called the senior strategy "*Mis Mejores Años*" ("My Best Years").

In his inauguration speech, he outlined his promises and expectations of the people. The spirit of the nation was crucial to the man who recognized humor as essential to well-being.

> The main and most important thing is I expect you to be happy.

Concerned for the welfare of all, in one public address, President Moreno commented on advances in Ecuadorian society.

> For too long, the disabled were ignored. Don't forget, there was a time when disabilities were

considered illnesses. Disabilities were also considered a punishment from God. People with mental challenges were considered demonic. They were the outcasts of the outcasts. They were denied any possibility of social connections. They were hidden and shunned.

These forgotten minorities were not small in number. According to President Moreno, there were a billion people in the world with some form of disability, making it the largest minority on the planet. At the time of his presidency, the country of Ecuador, which is smaller than the state of Nevada, registered 420,000 people with disabilities.

I should say, with great satisfaction, that our country is [now] the most advanced when it comes to promoting the rights of the disabled.

For example, one program he instituted tapped into a health promoter network to infiltrate even the most remote areas and determine the needs of, and find solutions for, the differently abled. President Moreno said the Manuelas, as the outreach workers were called:

...shined a light on the disabled community. The whole country took part. This [disabled] society regained its dignity. Because when society raises awareness for people with disabilities, it is not the person with the disability who regains his or her dignity, but the sad society that was keeping them in the dark.

The disabled reflect the diversity in humans, and diversity is beautiful. Speaking about his beloved country, President Moreno proudly shared:

We have diversity in climate, in topography, in biology, even in the way people dress, in our language, our customs, folklore and historic facts—and also among human beings. At birth, some people may be labeled differently abled compared to others who may be considered fully abled. But that is not correct. The term "disabled" does not define someone. We really have no proper term to define us. A small child may not be able to reach up to change a light bulb or, because of lack of coordination, a youngster cannot tie his or her shoelaces, [but we do not call them disabled]. Diversity. Diversity.

The Guru's Wisdom: Laugh Away Your Pain

One of President Moreno's favorite poems is about a child's laughter. The poet Miguel Hernandez was a Franco regime political prisoner. He died in jail at the age of thirty-one without ever holding or hugging his second son. The poet imagines that his boy's contagious laughter gives him the wings to break free from jail. Specifically, the child's laughter soothes the father's solitude and forges his sword of victory. Laughter is the most powerful tool, according to the poet and President Moreno.

We are the only species that can provoke or respond with laughter. Babies laugh long before they can talk. It is normal for children in their first few years of life to laugh often. But as they get older, they learn to hold back the instinct. Too often, adults tell them, "Don't laugh. This is serious." And children follow orders and disconnect that natural healing switch. Former President Moreno believes when children are taught to always be serious, they lose the ability to enjoy life to the fullest.

In the olden days, Ecuadorian women were not allowed to laugh. While men roared with laughter, women had to suppress their instincts behind a closed mouth, a symbol of their repression.

On the other side of the world, as recently as 1996, the Taliban outlawed public laughter for women in Afghanistan. During that regime, which obliterated the rights of females, 97 percent of women experienced major depression.

Without a doubt, it was laughter that brought Lenín Moreno up from the darkness. Laughter gave him what narcotics could not. It dulled his persistent pain and brought him a renewed love for life. He became entrenched in the topic of laughter, buying every book and movie he could find about the subject. He connected online with humorists. The former president became such a proponent of, and expert on, humor that he created laughter conferences where he lectured on risoterapia, and he even considered opening a comedy club.

President Moreno understands that humor abounds in an imperfect world. Since the world will never be perfect, we need to tap into lightheartedness to brighten our lives. The best jokes are byproducts of the most serious of times.

As a paraplegic, he battled unexpected prejudices, conflicts and barriers after his assault. He was no longer the strong, active, dignified man he had always been. His mobility was reliant on a wheelchair. He could not kick a soccer ball with his grandchildren or play tennis with his wife. However, what he had lost was made up for with extra compassion and the determination to make a difference for the physically and mentally challenged and the population as a whole.

In 2007, then-Vice President Moreno welcomed Hunter "Patch" Adams,[35] founder and director of the Gesundheit! Institute, to Ecuador and honored him with a solidarity medal of honor. Both men wore red clown noses.

Four years later, Dr. Adams returned to Ecuador to support "*Sonríe* (Smile) Ecuador," one of the vice president's national initiatives to encourage optimism, faith and laughter. Standing next to Dr. Adams, then-Vice President Moreno accused society of using chemicals and drugs to give ourselves a boost of positivity, when all we really need are a few hardy laughs.

> You just need to experience it. Humor helps people reflect on what is important and that is to enjoy life fully. I've confirmed the medicinal strength of humor. I have verified that humor has not only medicinal but immunological and therapeutic effects. It prevents illnesses as well as cures them.[36]

In 2014, the Maison de l'Humour de Cluny (House of Laughter and Humor) in Cluny, France, honored then-Vice President Moreno with the *L'Humour de Résistance* award for overcoming obstacles with a sense of humor. The Ecuadorian politician said:

> I relate to humor because it is such an important facet to human beings.[37]

Humans are not healthy if they shut out humor. The adage "you are what you eat" extends beyond the contents of your plate to your frame of mind, according to the former president.

> A healthy community lives happily and can build educated, creative, friendly and productive families. We have to abandon those habits that wounded our physical, mental and spiritual states of being. Sometimes we have to free ourselves from toxic thoughts and feelings. They are

> very harmful and can make us sicker, possibly even more than our diet... It is important to teach our children not only to eat nutritious food but to release toxic thoughts, emotions, feelings or memories and not be a slave to the toxicity. Be the loving owner of your thoughts and delight in positive habits.

According to President Moreno, there are two major contributing factors to how people embrace or deflect happiness. One factor is about basic needs like food, clothing, shelter, employment, family and health. The second, and more important, contributor to happiness is our subjective responses to how we enjoy life. Not everyone can have the dream job, house, vacation or partner. There is no exact correlation between money or health and happiness. The main variable is appreciation and contentment. We can all gain a sense of thankfulness for wherever we work and live, and with whomever and whatever surrounds our daily lives. Too often, people worry about the past or the future. The answer is to enjoy each moment.

Understanding the laws of quantum physics increased President Moreno's appreciation of humor as a significant part of life.

> Quantum physics is just the scientific explanation for spirituality. We are only an illusion. Matter is just an illusion. Time is just an illusion. Matter is just a construct of the mind that enables us to interpret this planetary soup. The world is not real. It is *maya*, an illusion. So just enjoy it.[38]

He joked during a Maison de l'Humour interview about two quantum physicists. The first physicist learned that a scientist from another lab discovered a subatomic particle. He was conflicted. He was elated with the discovery but disappointed that the breakthrough was not his. When asked how he felt about the discovery he said, "More or less like if you saw your mother-in-law falling off a cliff, but in your Ferrari."[39]

The quantum physics fan often peppered his official addresses with quotes from people as diverse as the theoretical physicist and cosmologist Stephen Hawking, characters from Indigenous folktales, the Bible and modern-day authors.

During one speech, he quoted the Chinese philosopher Lao Tse. "To lead people, walk behind them." To illustrate the point, he spoke about the former president of Venezuela, General Carlos Soublette. Soublette learned that there was a stage play poking fun at him. He called the author and said, "Sir, I know you are working on a piece called 'His Most Excellence' in which I'm laughed at."

"That's correct, Mr. President," said the playwright.

Soublette asked if he could see the play and the playwright nervously agreed. The president viewed the performance and laughed without restraint.

Shocked, the dramatist asked, "Mr. President, can we present this play where the public laughs at you?"

Soublette's response was, "The country will not suffer because the people laugh at an elected official. The harm is when the government laughs at the people."

Former President Moreno's Five Easy Tips

1. Be happy.

   Change your attitude and you change your life. Our mood defines us. Don't let it overshadow day-to-day problems. Counter unhappiness with active, respectful, friendly, supportive participation. Hatred wounds and causes pain. In the end, hatred only harms the one that holds on to it.

2. **Love what you are doing.**
   The greatest time for intellectual and innovative productiveness is not when you are working or studying, but when you are having fun. When you go for a walk or take a stroll, your mind begins to solve your unresolved problems from when you were at work or studying hard. Break from the doldrums. Go to a concert or a museum, or do something else you find uplifting.

3. **Choose the biggest fight: better yourself.**
   There is no one to improve but yourself, and you have to do the work on your own.

4. **Erase failure from your vocabulary.**
   True failure is doing nothing. If you fail after you have tried, you always have another chance to learn from the experience and improve the next time around. Never let failures hold you back.

5. **Open up to the glories surrounding you.**
   The beauty of being human is that we can perceive not only colors, forms and textures, but scents, flavors and even the spirit of our ancestral warriors. Awaken your senses to appreciate what's around you.

Laughter on Call

It is human nature to laugh. The natural process is healthy for our bodies and our souls. The art of comedy is not natural for everyone, including me. But as a certified Laughter Yoga Leader,

I can elicit laughter for twenty to forty minutes at a time with no jokes.

I first experienced laughter yoga in Varanasi, India, as part of a traditional holistic yoga session conducted in Hindi. I was sitting on the ground under a large tent with about one hundred women wearing saris or tunic-like *kurtas*. The men sat elsewhere. I squeezed in at the end of a row next to a frail and timid-looking younger woman who did not speak English. For close to an hour, she stared at me as if I was an alien. I tried to send her a smile, but her dourness didn't change. For the last five or ten minutes of class, we were instructed to force out huge belly laughs and point at each other. With no one on my other side, I zoomed in on the lady with the snarly attitude. I got such a kick out of doing this that our fake snickers turned into honest-to-goodness, seriously unstoppable laughter. Little by little, it tore down whatever walls were between us. When we left, I felt energized by her friendly eyes and smile. Laughter was the lingua franca and the dopamine-producing tonic that had me floating away in a great mood.

In laughter yoga, they say "fake it until you make it." Dr. Madan Kataria first introduced Laughter Clubs in a Mumbai park in 1995, not to entertain, but to heal. When his bevy of jokes ran dry, he realized that simulated laughter would have an equal impact on the body and the brain. Then, his wife added 4,000-year-old yogic breathing techniques to stimulate the parasympathetic nervous system, simple movement to expand the diaphragm, and playfulness to release inhibitions. The result was laughter yoga, which is an aerobic practice that focuses on simulated diaphragmatic laughter and is appropriate for most people, young or old.[40] Participants agree their emotional, physical and spiritual health is significantly better, and they are even laughing more outside of the sessions. Now there are twenty thousand free Laughter Yoga clubs in one hundred twenty countries. In India, they meet every day and also serve as a network for positive social interaction.

Shortly after my introduction to Dr. Kataria's invention, I met LaBet Pritchard. I attended one of her laughter yoga classes with my psychotherapist daughter and her social worker friend. We knew it would be amusing and an hour of unofficial professional development for each of us.

LaBet agrees with Lenín Moreno.

> Laughter is a miracle drug. It increases the endorphins, serotonin, dopamine and oxytocin in the brain and is especially effective in a group since the connection made through eye contact stimulates the mirror neurons of the brain. These feel-good hormones are contagious. Even when alone, as evidenced by Dr. Norman Cousins in his 1979 autobiography, *Anatomy of an Illness,* laughing at *The Three Stooges* movies in an empty hotel room can cure life-threatening disease.

Most noticeable is the immediate release of tension. The body is relaxed. The mind is no longer replaying fears about tomorrow's deadlines. Laughter reduces inhibitions while boosting our natural senses of creativity and positivity. Not as obvious, belly laughter tones the abdominal muscles and fine-tunes facial expressions.

LaBet witnessed a wide range of positive effects from the practice. "Laughter is the best medicine. It sure worked to cure most of what has ever ailed me."

Not long after LaBet completed her initial yoga teacher training, she heard about a three-day laughter yoga intensive. "What do I do, but jump a plane to Los Angeles and laugh my ass off?" Her face was sore from the unsuppressed smiles and laughter, but the real benefits were far beneath the skin.

It was just about the weirdest thing I have ever done. It seemed to trigger and uncover some deeply buried trauma and emotional baggage that it was time to face. I was an alcoholic in an unhappy marriage and seemed to think booze and laughter were going to heal my miserable situation.

Over the next two years, I left my marriage, went to rehab, joined Alcoholics Anonymous, and surrendered to a new way of life. I faced my fears. I stepped through the threshold equipped with the newly found confidence to teach just about anything—sober. I stretched myself by teaching yoga with a bit of laughter sprinkled in here and there. People loved it. They were amazed at how lighthearted, joyful and jovial they felt at the end of class. I went on to take my 500-hour [advanced] yoga therapy training and focused on yoga and the twelve steps with a lot of humor interspersed.

There is scientific evidence to explain what LaBet, President Moreno, and people around the world have experienced. Laughing releases endorphins, which are natural opiates that mimic the pain-numbing effects of morphine.[41] Plus, the act of prolonged laughter increases circulation and oxygenation, strengthens the lungs, and protects the heart.

During my laughter yoga training, we learned about Dr. Lee Berk at the Loma Linda University Medical Center, who says joyful laughter builds the body's immune system by increasing antibodies and T-cell activity.[42]

Dr. Berk also researched high-risk diabetic patients with hypertension and found that those who practiced laughter therapy for a year had better vital signs, decreased stress indicators and improved HDL cholesterol.[43]

In addition, laughter yoga uses role-playing and pantomiming to heighten appreciation and forgiveness.

The resulting changes in our brains can be beneficial too. The amygdala and hippocampus (responsible for emotions, anxiety, learning and memory) are activated as a response to something funny. Listening to slapstick or faking it until you make it reduces stress hormones, slows the aging process, and brings back the playful, carefree child.

Developmental and neuropsychology researchers in Europe conducted a systemic review and meta-analysis of laughter-inducing therapies.[44] Their findings propose that simulated laughter is more effective than spontaneous outbreaks for combating depression, pain, stress and mood disorders. The methods the researchers explored for simulating and stimulating laughter included solo or group clapping, dancing, facial exercises, watching clowns, and laughter exercises, all of which are elements of laughter yoga.

Give It a Try:
Laugh Out Loud!

There are unlimited ways to bring laughter into your life. Rather than tuning in to violent action-packed programs or movies, choose something cheerful and amusing. Within your social media world, find, follow, share or repost funny memes rather than glum or woe-is-me reports. Take ten to fifteen minutes out of your day to laugh, even if you are by yourself with nothing funny in sight.

1. **Shout Ho-Ho-Ho.**

   Set a timer to sixty seconds. Once it starts, walk around as if you are Santa Claus on Christmas Eve. With every exhalation, in a very loud and low voice, shout "ho-ho-ho." Let your inner child out as you mimic the sound of deep laughter from the gut. Focus on the belly and the breath. Clap or pound a fist at the sky with each sound. When your timer is done, take a few slow deep breaths in and out through your nose. Feel the difference in your body and your mind.

2. **Titter Tee-Hee-Hee.**

   Set your timer for one or two minutes. Instead of the big bulky Santa, now you are as tiny as Tinker Bell, the pixie in Peter Pan. With every exhalation, fold forward with knees bent (only if you don't have osteoporosis, osteopenia or high blood pressure). Light as a butterfly, playfully laugh "tee-hee-hee." Simultaneously, visualize something hilarious as you giggle.

3. **Take a trip.**

   Aloha. Imagine you just landed in Hawaii. With the first breath, reach your arms up, palms facing forward as you say "Ahhh. Low." On the second exhalation, swing the arms down with a long extended "ha-ha-ha." Repeat five or six times or more—unless you want to stay on the island longer.

In short, sometimes you need to release the burdens that weigh you down and revert to carefree, childlike play. Laughter is one of the most natural and healthy instincts.

The next suggestion is singing, which you were introduced to as a baby. And it should be just as enjoyable now.

Chapter 4: Singing and Silence Bring Inner Peace

There was a little girl
who held for the world
a vision no one understood.
Love, peace and harmony.
She said her prayers at night
and knew one day she just might
realize her dream.
Love, peace and harmony.
Love wide as the blue sky.

—Randall Brooks, "Blue Sky"

B hakti is my favorite form of yoga, hands down. It's not about the body, but about the heart. *Bhakti* may be best described as devotion and can be expressed by singing, chanting, drumming or tuning in to silence.

My travel plans are influenced by bhakti gatherings from Costa Rica to India. At the yoga studio, my Spotify preferences are set to *kirtan*, the spiritual call-and-response music associated with bhakti yoga. I've even curated more than one hundred kirtan-infused playlists, including selections from the Bhakti House Band, led by Randall and Kristin Brooks.

I first met the couple at the Texas Yoga Conference in Houston in 2015. A few dozen of us crowded onto an elevated schoolhouse stage with open proscenium curtains overlooking the conference expo center as we chanted 108 rounds of the Gayatri mantra.

This mantra, which dates back three thousand years, is an invocation of light, peace and healing. "Gayatri" is the name of the goddess who imparts light in our minds, which correlates to the word "guru," meaning "remover of darkness" (which is light). As with most mantras, tradition holds that you chant 108 repetitions.

The Brookses led the vocals and played harmonium[45] and percussion, while one of their bandmates created a soothing undercurrent with a bevy of wind chimes and singing bowls. The vibrations of the instruments and the chanting enveloped me as we sat on the hard wooden floor.

Having studied five foreign languages in college, I find Sanskrit easy to pronounce. However, Randall and Kristin's attention to the subtle nuances of the ancient language made it clear my interpretation of some sounds was far off. The linguist in me, coupled with my love for bhakti yoga, led me to spend more time with the Brookses. Over the next five years, I joined the couple chanting kirtan on sizable stages from California to Wisconsin.

On March 1, 2020, I chatted with Randall and Kristin at a bhakti festival in Dallas. Two weeks later, the coronavirus pandemic hit and quarantines eliminated live performances. In response, the devotional singers launched the Bhakti House Café, online daily sessions filled with uplifting words and spiritual music. For more than a year, we stayed connected via their virtual *satsang* (sacred gathering of truth).

A House Full of Bhakti: Randall and Kristin Brooks

Randall and Kristin Brooks are professional musicians and *bhaktas* (individuals dedicated to a life of devotion). As masters of sacred sound as well as ancient scriptures and languages, they like to say that their home is their ashram. Long ago, they dubbed their Fort Worth residence the "Bhakti House" and invited people to be a part of making music there, giving rise to the award-winning Bhakti House Band.

Randall is a rapper and the rebellious son of a Southern Baptist preacher. He studied Aramaic, Greek, Hebrew and San-skrit to be able to deconstruct sacred texts. He found the Bible, both the Old and New Testaments, mirrored yogic messages and perspectives.

Kristin comes from a family of doctors and was raised in the wealthy part of Fort Worth. But she was not your normal kid with a teddy bear.

> At age two, I told my mom I was going to be pres-
> ident of the world and preach love on big stages.
> From the time I could walk, I wanted nothing
> more than to swing on my swing set and sing
> with God all day long.

Music was her life and connection to her soul. She studied classical piano and voice and performed in Broadwayesque musicals. Artistic expression was also her refuge since Kristin had been a victim of multiple violent crimes and was what she calls "the queen of abusive relationships." She found solace in the Bible verse, "Seek ye first the kingdom of God, and his righteousness; and all these things shall be added unto you."

(Matthew 6:33 KJV) That simple rule changed everything for her once she prioritized her relationship with the divine.

The day Kristin met Randall, she knew they were meant to create love, peace and harmony together. He is the main singer and songwriter. She is the pianist and adds melodic overtones. Both play harmonium and *dholak* (a two-headed Indian hand drum). Their percussion-driven music blends East and West through rhythms and vocals. In their eclectic style, they mix English and Sanskrit, rap, rock and gospel folk with classical Indian music. To carry out their pledge to spread love, peace and light, they encourage listeners to let go of the external chaos and surrender to the rhythmic groove of the heart.

In fact, their devotion to music and the divine was their saving grace when Randall and Kristin nearly lost their third and youngest child. They had a planned home delivery, but there were complications. Baby Fen was not breathing after his birth and was in fetal distress.

The midwife gave mouth-to-mouth resuscitation until little Fen gasped for air. Just when they thought they were in the clear, their baby turned grayish-blue. They rushed to a nearby hospital, which was ill-equipped, so a pediatric transport team shuttled the newborn to a medical center an hour away. Randall and Kristin sang spiritual songs during the trip to remain positive. When they got to the second hospital, a preacher walked up to them and proclaimed, "This baby shall not die, but he shall live."

Things were looking grim. Fen was in critical condition. His oxygen saturation levels dipped to the 30s. (The optimum is 100.) Meconium (fetal waste) and blood clogged up his lungs. Sepsis from strep pneumonia and E. *coli* bacteria ravaged their baby. Finally, he was transferred to a third hospital with an even better neonatal intensive care unit (NICU).

Kristin recalls:

> We got there in the middle of the night. After hours, the doctor came into the waiting room and sat down. That's never a good sign. He said, "You need to start thinking about preparations because he will not make it through the night."
>
> At that moment, divine energy calmed me. I knew my baby was in the best care possible. We decided to move to that higher level of consciousness.

Baby Fen did survive the night. However, he was in critical condition for weeks. Precautionary measures restricted the parents from holding or touching their baby, except on rare occasions.

At the same time, Randall and Kristin needed their own protection from the barrage of negativity. Another callous doctor told them, "I'm leaving for the weekend. I probably won't see you again. There's nothing more I can do. By the time I come back, your baby will be gone."

They tuned out the insensitivity and the gloomy prognosis on Fen's chart. The couple continued to project a positive outcome for their baby. In the meantime, they wrote a detailed picture of Fen's homecoming in their dream journal and committed their hearts and minds to that story, regardless of what the medical staff insisted.

Back at home during a respite from the hospital, Randall and Kristin once again got news that Fen was not going to make it. A nurse had called and told them to come to say goodbye to their baby. Driving to the hospital, they redirected the pain with the lyrics of one of their favorite pop/R&B songs by Natasha Bedingfield, "Unwritten."

As they sang, they saw positive signs all around them. Kristin reflected on the moment.

> Etched in my mind forever was the sunrise coming up. Yellows and oranges and purples and pinks brilliantly covered the entire panorama like somebody turned the saturation of the colors all the way up. A feeling of well-being came over me. I knew there was nothing that could separate me from my son.
>
> When we got to the NICU, it was like one of those angel moments. There was this maintenance guy working there. Never saw him before. Never saw him after. And there he was with his tiny transistor radio playing Natasha Bedingfield's song "Unwritten."

Kristin took it as an omen. When they arrived at Fen's bedside, there was a daunting cluster of thirty or forty doctors and nurses. The head nurse told Randall and Kristin, "We can't explain it. It's a miracle." Fen was suddenly on the road to recovery.

It was at that moment when the couple realized the power of clear intention and deep surrender of devotion.

> However you want to call it: divine love, Christ consciousness, Buddha consciousness, Krishna consciousness... It's that real connection to the divine—that true experience of one-ness. Dance with the universe. Release resistance. Any obstacle is the opportunity to expand one's awareness.

The Gurus' Wisdom: Sing to Heal

Besides being full-time kirtan musicians, the Brookses teach nada yoga (union through sacred sound, vibration or cosmic music).

That may seem a bit intangible, but Kristin and her husband are not "airy-fairy." Underneath the singing, strumming and spreading light and love in devotion, they are grounded. They dig deep into the wisdom of scientists, spiritualists and sages and teach and preach from a base of accepted practice.

In describing their method, Kristin explains:

> Singing produces endorphins and oxytocin and turns off the part of the brain that tells us we are separate. Singing with others opens the heart, encourages community bonding, and develops authentic and intimate friendships more quickly than any other activity. Science tells us that everything is vibration. We are vibration. We are living music. Sound healing is just natural vibrational healing.

For those who practice kirtan, there is often an extended pause between chants to feel the vibrations within. Randall and Kristin treasure the blissful space between the songs. Those sounds of silence are a powerful form of meditation or tuning in. The quiet gives the practitioner time to soak up the moment, almost like savasana, the final relaxation at the end of a physical yoga session.

Kristin encourages listeners to let go of the external chaos and surrender their minds to the rhythmic groove within.

> The power of sound in movement leads us to the even greater power of sound in stillness. The

sound of silence, the inner om, is the unstruck song of the heart, where we experience our true power.

When I feel lost, I return to the inner music, or as the ancients, sages and mystics called it, the *nadam* (the first vibration). It is in the *anahata* (heart) nadam where I find my rest. The closer we stay to that refuge within, the more pure the love is in our lives. Things vibrate from within, outward. Think of it as your heart exploding. A love bomb. A truth bomb.

That's why the yoga of sacred sound helps us to connect within ourselves and with others. Just like there are many genres of music and ways to meditate, there is no one right way to practice nada yoga. The only requisite is to release extraneous thoughts and let your heart and soul take over.

Chanting mantras, singing, clapping, playing instruments, or dancing—all of which are second nature to young children—can help you get to that sweet spot of the silence within.

Play a recorded song or mantra that calms you. Then close your eyes, take a few centering breaths, and sing or move to the rhythm. When you come to a pause, soak up the silent vibrations. In some traditions, ecstatic dancing is a part of bhakti, whereas in others, praying is accompanied by a gentle rocking back and forth. Movements that connect the mind, body and spirit are forms of yoga and are positive, conscious and efficient ways to spend your energy.

Kristin says:

Through music, I feel and experience love. Love drives me to live. We all have an entry point to experiencing the divine, or God, depending on our upbringing, our culture, our religion, or our personal experience. The way our individual nature translates the energy of our relationship with the divine is going to be different for everyone. When we engage our voice in song, we engage our creative nature and cultivate our connection to the divine.

Randall continues:

Chanting turns off the part of the brain that tells us we're separate, so we connect with others. These sacred mantras, like the Gayatri, have been chanted for thousands of years, and we're connecting back [to prior generations] through that lineage of light.

You can chant, sing or move to the beat in any language or using any instrument.

All cultures throughout time have had forms of sacred music and names for the Creator. Around the world, there are nearly one thousand names people use for God. In Islam, there are ninety-nine expressions for God. Kabbalah counts seventy-two monikers. The Hindu[46] Vaishnavas[47] say there are unlimited labels for the Supreme Being. All are reflections of the one God and all are holy names. No one form is better or worse, which is why many who practice bhakti yoga will refer to the holy name using a variety of expressions.

As the rap bridge in the Bhakti House Band's song, "Blue Sky" says:

In my father's house are many rooms
with Christian, Hindu, Jain and Jew,
Muslim, Sikh and all other blooms.
But there's only one behind the costumes.

Randall encourages people to practice in any style and language they choose.

> Do your best. Then later on, when you let yourself
> go with the flow, the pronunciation will take form.
> We always say in chanting Sanskrit, it's devotion
> first. Just open your heart and feel, and it will do
> its work.

It doesn't matter if you understand the words. People pray in Latin, Hebrew and Arabic, often without understanding the language. Sanskrit is a celestial language that can be associated with multiple philosophies and religions, including Hinduism, Jainism[48] and Buddhism.

According to Kristin:

> Sanskrit's ability to organize sound into a precise
> alphabet of infinite potential, along with rules of
> grammar that cover every possible form of man-
> ifestation and expression, allows us to remove
> any unnecessary fluff we tend to find in many
> modern languages. It cuts to the chase. Sanskrit
> organizes the cosmic music into a beautifully
> efficient, poetic song, yet leaves nothing out and
> accounts for all infinite possibilities making up
> our ever-expanding "uni-verse" or "one song."

That is also why it is difficult to translate Sanskrit. More often than not, one word in English does not express the Sanskrit meaning.

The word "Sanskrit" means "perfection." Each letter in its alphabet is a *bija*, or seed mantra, tiny yet with unlimited potential. The most well-known of all the Sanskrit bijas is "om." With repetition, the bijas create balance and energy. There is a seed mantra to correspond to each of the seven primary chakras or energetic centers that rise from the base of the spine to the crown of the head.

Always trying to share their positive mindset, Kristin says:

There's a lot of crap in the world. Use it as fertilizer.

A single seed holds all the information and essence of a fully manifested forest. There's no need to chop all the trees down to start a new forest. A seed is simple and refined, yet carries infinite potential.

We are going to the sound vibrational level, underneath. We're shaking off whatever muck we're attached to, consciously tilling the ground and planting the seeds.

Give it a shot. Sow those seeds by practicing your mantras and watch what grows in your heart and soul. It is commonly believed that Confucius said:

Music produces a kind of pleasure which human nature cannot do without.

Randall and Kristin Brookses' Five Easy Tips

1. Sing every day.
   Sing in the shower, in the car, at church or during yoga and notice the improvement in your mood. Exercise your vocal chords with your dog, kids, parents or friends. When we raise our voice in song, we engage our creative nature and cultivate our connection to the divine.

2. Become childlike in your creativity and quest for learning.
   Make life an adventure and play it as if it's a game you just cannot lose. Have fun without self-judgment. Relish how good the freedom of expression feels.

3. **Serve and uplift humanity with your talents, abilities and gifts.**

    Use your God-given gifts to serve others. Service inspires and reinforces communal connections while keeping us from becoming hyperfocused on ourselves.

4. **Release negative emotions.**

    Establish yourself in peace, compassion and love in accordance with yoga's first commandment: *ahimsa* (do no harm). Follow the nonviolence principles of Mahatma Gandhi and Dr. Martin Luther King, Jr., the latter of whom said, "Darkness cannot drive out darkness; only light can do that. Hate cannot drive out hate; only love can do that."[49]

5. **Love yourself and love others.**

    Make an extra effort to be patient and kind with yourself and everyone around you. Patanjali's [50] *Yoga Sutras* remind us to cultivate an attitude of friendliness toward those who are happy, show compassion for the suffering, express joyful celebration to the virtuous, and be nonjudgmental of those who appear to be doing evil.

The Feel-Good Hormones

Some of my dearest childhood memories are linked to music. But there was no training, beyond maybe a year of piano lessons and a few months lugging around a three-time hand-me-down clarinet. I have zero recollection of ever producing any pleasant sounds from that old thing, but I remember the feel of the smooth, cool, cane reeds on my lips.

There wasn't much music in my house. My mom liked quiet. When she was working away from home, I ate lunch at her friend's house. A radio always played in the background in their kitchen. The station rotated mellow songs from the '60s. As I ate—most often grilled cheese and tomato soup—I heard my mom's friend singing along in a clear and confident voice to Barbra Streisand or Eydie Gormé. Joy radiated throughout her home.

I never paid much attention to lyrics or instrumentation. It was just the vocals that I heard and felt.

Sunday mornings, while everyone else at my house was still asleep, I would head down to the family room. Perched on top of a red-and-white checkered tablecloth was our only television. It was a black-and-white set with rabbit ear antennae and a dial to select between the only five channels with programming. Of course, these were the days before cable or remote control.

During church time, the queen of gospel, Mahalia Jackson, sang a few feet away from me, through that bulky console. Her voice and inner fire were captivating. The power and devotion in her songs of praise were nothing like the squawking band or dishwatery chorus classes at my predominantly White elementary school.

Even better than listening to Mahalia on the tube was singing with my older sister in our living room to an invisible audience from a make-believe stage on our green, low-pile carpeted floor. We harmonized to *The Sound of Music* and *Mary Poppins*. At those moments, I was in heaven.

In 1970, my sister bought her first LP, The 5th Dimension's *Greatest Hits*. Singing along to "Stoned Soul Picnic," "Wedding Bell Blues," and "Let The Sun Shine In" was a rush. The songs reverberated. I experienced nada yoga without knowing what hit me.

More than thirty years later, I found the nada again at Swami Sita's ashram in California. (You'll meet her in "Chapter 10: Serving is the Secret of Abundance.") After that, I was determined to keep bhakti yoga in my normal routine. Chanting devotional songs brought me back to those natural highs I felt as a kid.

Today, my daily bhakti practices include several styles. Every morning and at bedtime, I whisper mantras almost on autopilot for about an hour. Whenever I want to be more energized, I turn up my volume and sing kirtan by myself to the recordings of my favorite bhakti musicians like the Bhakti House Band. I also regularly attend a group kirtan for full spiritual and sensory bliss.

Don Campbell, in his book *The Mozart Effect*, says:

> In an instant, music can uplift our soul. Music can dance and sing our blues away. The human voice is a remarkable instrument of healing, our most accessible sonic tool. The slightest utterance massages muscle tissue in the upper body and causes it to vibrate from within.[51]

Research confirms that singers have lower cortisol levels, meaning they are less stressed out. Chanting or singing, like breathwork, activates the parasympathetic system, thereby lowering blood pressure and producing a Zen-like state.

Remember Julie Andrews and her seven frightened kids in *The Sound of Music*? They all huddled in the governess's bedroom during a thunderstorm. By the time they finished singing "My Favorite Things," the children didn't "feel so bad." The magic of music is not just a Rodgers and Hammerstein fairy tale. It is a science that helps us release those feel-good hormones.

One study from the University of Gothenburg in Sweden found that those who sang together had synchronized heartbeats. Singing is a form of controlled breathing, like yoga, and research has shown that heart rate variability (HRV) and respiration affect each other, with slow respiration producing higher HRV amplitudes.[52]

The same study also evaluated the effect on the heart rate of humming a single tone, singing a Christian hymn, or repeating the mantra "just relax." While humming had its benefits, the hymn and mantra had a greater effect on heart rate variability.

Furthermore, singing also affects heart-brain coherence and HRV, or the measurement of spacing between each heartbeat. Over many years, research has shown a definite relationship between low HRV and depression, anxiety and cardiovascular disease. The variability slows down with mindfulness, meditation, sleep and music, which correlates to elevated moods.

A smaller study in Italy contrasted singing "Ave Maria" with chanting the mantra "om mani padme om."[53] Both practices showed improved HRV.

Praising all varieties of music, sound and humming, Campbell says in The Mozart Effect:

> Music can drum out evil spirits, sing the praises of the Virgin Mary, invoke the Buddha of the Universal Salvation, enchant leaders and nations, captivate and soothe, resurrect and transform.

Give It a Try:
Tuning Your Chakras

If you're not familiar with the chakras, here is a list of each of them, along with their associated location within your body, as well as their bija and color. Feel free to consult this page until you have memorized the locations, bijas and colors for each or download a colorful chakra poster from my website at deborahcharnes.com/chakras.

Chakra	Location	Bija	Color
First	base of the spine	lam	red
Second	below the navel	vam	orange
Third	solar plexus	ram	yellow
Fourth	heart	yam	green
Fifth	throat	ham	blue
Sixth	third eye	om	indigo
Seventh	crown	ah-oo-mm-ng	violet or white

Repeating simple one-syllable bija (seed) mantras is a powerful practice for the mind, body and spirit. The Brookses lead and practice these exercises at least once a week. To see a video of them walking you through a bija mantra, visit deborahcharnes.com/bija.

1. **Sit comfortably.**
   Lengthen your spine and relax the shoulders. Let your chin hang gently. Imagine the crown of your head reaching to the sky. Relax.

2. **Inhale through the nose and exhale through the mouth.**
   With each inhalation, focus on the word "inhale."

With each exhalation, silently say "exhale." Fill up your lungs and squeeze out the air to release toxins.

3. **Focus on each chakra, one at a time.**

As you continue breathing through your mouth, focus on the location and color of each chakra as you chant its associated bija. Repeat each bija out loud, trying to connect from one to the next. Start with the first chakra and continue for a full minute. Then one by one repeat the process until you've reached the last chakra.

4. **Inhale as needed, but try to repeat the bija as many times as possible with one exhalation.**

Feel the buzzing of the consonants in your sinuses and throughout your body (especially the final /m/, which is nasalized like /ng/) and visualize the associated color and area for each chakra.

5. **When you get to the crown chakra, visualize a lotus floating just above your head.**

This time, instead of repeating one syllable for a minute, break up each of the sounds found within "om." With each long exhalation, try to extend each of the four sounds: /a/, /oo/, /m/, /ng/. Continue as long as you like.

6. **When done, place one or two hands over your heart and focus on the connection between the palm and the heart.**

As Kristin says, "Feel how the bija seeds have begun to sprout." This practice tends to generate peace of mind and body.

After applying the tips for mindfulness, yoga, laughter and chanting, you should feel as if you're floating on a cloud. Now it's time to focus on your body.

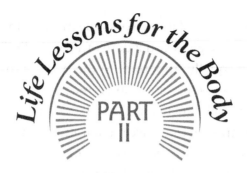

Life Lessons for the Body

PART
II

Everything is Connected

E very body is different, and everything inside us is connected. Little in life works in isolation. The medical community now agrees that the body and mind work in unison.
Aches are not always just physical. Diet, digestion, stress, mobility and other factors play a part.

Too often, we focus on one problem without seeing the big
picture. We take an aspirin for a headache without question-
ing why we are in pain. For a runny nose, we swallow an antihistamine that knocks us out. Or we choose the cough syrup
with caffeine to stay awake. The quick fix often hurts us in the
long run.

Think of it as a set of dominoes. If one piece falls, the rest
tumble down. Yet, if each component has a strong foundation and supports the other, it can withstand most jostles
and shake-ups.

When we think about our bodies, some actions and reactions are easy to grasp. For example, if we break a leg, the bones
need to reset. If we have a major cut, we need to stop the bleed-
ing. While drinking two liters of water is healthy, bottle after
bottle of beer is not. Spending the day watching television has
a different effect than gardening. Pulling weeds and mowing

the lawn boosts circulation, works the muscles and the joints, and if it is sunny gives you a dose of vitamin D. What is less obvious, but equally important to the body, is that the yard work immerses you in nature and is meditative.

The emotional benefits may not be tangible, but they are powerful. A stress-free positive mental attitude may be hard to measure, but the body (and spirit) can feel the difference.

Many spiritual traditions liken the body to clothing. Our skin and bones only cover up our true identity: our soul. Ancient wisdom teaches that our body changes every day. The person in the last stages of their life bears little resemblance to when they were a toddler.

On a cellular level, we are also in a nonstop state of flux. We cannot bring back lost hair or reverse graying without chemicals or hair dye. But just as a weight lifter can build muscles, we can change the physical. With different habits, intentions and even frames of mind, we can alter our bodies on many levels. We can tone, fortify or nourish our bones, connective tissues, internal organs and nervous system through practices that are both visible and invisible.

Chapter 5: Backing Away from Back Pain

Yoga and arthritis were made for each other.

—Dr. Loren Fishman

I consider Loren Fishman, MD, the guru for bones, joints and the back: those parts that keep us moving, standing, walking and even sleeping. The educational offerings of the medical director of Manhattan Physical Medicine and Rehabilitation sparked my own therapeutic workshops for back and bone issues. I treasure soaking up whatever I can from experts like him who combine ancient Vedic[54] lessons and traditions with the stringent testing that's the norm in the modern medical field.

The curriculum vitae of this physiatrist (a physical structure expert) and professor at Columbia Medical School is about fifty pages long. Dr. Fishman has published a dozen books including *Yoga for Back Pain* and *Healing Yoga*. His research findings have been televised on ABC's *World News Tonight* with Diane Sawyer. Despite all his credentials, he comes across as a down-to-earth doctor who just wants to help people feel better.

My first encounter with Dr. Fishman was at an annual conference of the International Association of Yoga Therapists in California. Aware of his accomplishments, when I saw his name on the agenda, I signed up for all his workshops. Later, during the pandemic, he launched virtual weekly classes and a weekend retreat. Thanks to videoconferencing, it was a cinch to participate despite 1,800 miles of physical distance.

The Doctor in the Lotus Pose: Dr. Loren Fishman

In addition to his other professional roles, Dr. Fishman is a yoga therapist. He views yoga from an anatomical and medical perspective, while acknowledging the practice's emotional and spiritual benefits.

Based on his decades of research, Dr. Fishman encourages those suffering from neurological and musculoskeletal back pain to consider yoga exercises before drugs or surgery. But first, given the complexities and myriad origins of back pain, any proposed exercise routine should be discussed with a medical practitioner and a certified yoga therapist or physical therapist. What's prescriptive for one person can be detrimental to another.

Besides staying current on the science behind yoga, the doctor has done quite a bit of research himself—not just fact-finding among friends and family, but megastudies. He's evaluated and treated thousands of patients with sciatic pain in the last twenty years.

Dr. Fishman probably has more experience than anyone with straightening the spine for people with scoliosis and strengthening bones for those with osteoporosis, with no medications or surgery. In the first peer-reviewed trial on yoga for scoliosis, which he spearheaded, adolescents and adults practiced just one specific yoga pose to improve curvature of the spine an average of 40 percent.

He discovered his own fix for torn rotator cuffs while waiting for his surgeon's calendar to open up to mend his injured shoulder. What he stumbled upon was a miracle cure. He has since introduced more than one thousand people to his technique, with 90 percent reporting all pain disappeared after his simple yogic-inspired approach.[55]

Worldwide, approximately two hundred million women have some degree of bone loss,[56] and many cannot afford or access medical care. Those facts fuel Dr. Fishman's passion for finding and sharing uncomplicated, accessible, low-cost, low-risk remedies.

In one long-term study, he chronicled the effects of yoga among 741 participants with osteoporosis or osteopenia.[57] Ultimately, his analysis tallied more than one hundred fifty thousand hours of yoga practice over fifteen years. Most important, his long-term research confirmed that even bone mineral density can be rebuilt with appropriate yoga techniques.

While Dr. Fishman is an expert on a bevy of disorders, he has aided more than twenty thousand patients with lower back pain alone,[58] which is why we're focusing on back pain in this chapter. But first, let's take a look at the man behind the lab coat.

Raised in Chicago, he completed his undergrad degree at the University of Michigan—Ann Arbor during the 1960s. He crossed the Atlantic and earned an advanced degree from Oxford. Not ready to return to the States, he spent three years in India. While there, he trained with the legendary B. K. S. Iyengar in Pune in 1973.

Despite Dr. Fishman's many life changes, his master's teachings have been a constant. The doctor has maintained a daily personal yoga practice since the '70s, and professionally, he encourages using yoga poses as a form of alternative treatment. The kid from Chicago found one of his greatest mentors in Iyengar.

The eleventh of thirteen children and a sickly child, the Indian adept survived a severe influenza pandemic, malaria, tuberculosis, typhoid and malnutrition. Under the tutelage of Sri[59] Krishnamacharya, his brother-in-law and one of the highest regarded yoga therapists of all time,[60] Iyengar became strong and healthy. At fifty-four, this master could melt his body—and mind—into poses that only a few Westerners (like Fishman) could mimic. Iyengar continued to practice challenging deep backbends, arm balances and twists while in his nineties. Shortly before he died at the age of ninety-five, he said, "I will not run away from my practice because of the fear complex of old age."

Fishman didn't just focus on his flexibility and endurance on the mat. He noticed the correlation between people's dedication to the postures and overall well-being as a result of the Eastern practice. After learning about yoga—and life—he returned to Chicago and attended medical school at Rush Presbyterian St. Luke's. Eventually, he landed in New York as chief resident in the department of rehabilitation medicine at Albert Einstein College of Medicine in the Bronx. All the while, his medical mind was integrating yoga therapy into his treatment plans.

Dr. Fishman established Manhattan Physical Medicine and Rehabilitation in 1997. While he prescribed surgery and medications when appropriate, he found yoga was often an inexpensive long-lasting fix with no negative side effects.

This doctor takes after his guru. Born in 1940, Dr. Fishman is a poster child for why yoga is good for your body and mind.

He still looks like a teenager when he gets into a yoga pose. At the same time, he doesn't demand or expect the same from his patients. He suggests adaptations with props, like a chair or wall, even for those far younger than him.

The Guru's Wisdom: Get to the Source of the Pain

Most of us have felt aches or pains in our back at one time or another. In fact, back pain will affect eight out of ten people in their lifetime. As a result, Americans spend more than $50 billion a year on back pain treatment and remedies.[61] Furthermore, back pain is the most common type of pain complaint[62] and often interferes with our ability to be present and productive in the workplace.[63]

Despite all the warnings about addictions, overdoses and deaths from opioids, in 2017, a quarter of those with back pain resorted to opioids.[64] By 2020, 75 percent of drug overdose deaths involved these highly addictive pain-killers.[65] Clearly, something is wrong with our society or healthcare system.

Dr. Fishman says pain is the most common affliction people experience. A significant percentage of medical visits are pain-related. Narrowing that down further, nonspecific backache is the third most common reason patients visit doctors.[66]

Pain is unpleasant, colorless, weightless, invisible... But it is there. Sometimes you can pinpoint the spot; other times, the ache or throbbing is diffuse. Wherever and whenever it occurs, you cannot deny the discomfort. Even worse, pain does not operate in isolation. Instead, it saps energy and concentration and is a mood buster.

One study on chronic pain and depression acknowledged up to 85 percent of those with chronic pain also suffer from severe depression, which is one of the top three contributors to disease worldwide.[67] As discussed earlier, yoga is an effective and inexpensive aid for emotional distress.

Neither depression nor pain appears out of nowhere. Dr. Fishman says what is essential is to identify the root cause. A rash may be due to herpes zoster or to poison ivy, but these two causes require opposite treatments.

With pain, it is the same. Depending on its cause, the pain may need to be treated in different and even contrary ways. Dr. Fishman explains that pain is just a symptom, and there are innumerable reasons behind it.

> Pain is universal. But you can't treat pain. You must treat its cause. The most important thing is to diagnose it accurately.

Consider the longest nerve in the body: the sciatic nerve. Those suffering from sciatica feel pain that can spread down their leg. Yet the problem is in the back, not the leg. That radiating pain is just a symptom of multiple potential issues ranging from a sciatic nerve compressed by a herniated disc, spinal stenosis,[68] spondylolisthesis[69] or piriformis syndrome.[70] Each condition requires a different treatment.

Unfortunately, it is not always easy to detect the root cause of pain. While anatomical variances, like uneven hips, scoliosis, kyphosis[71] or lordosis,[72] are pretty clear in a postural exam, oftentimes, even imaging like MRIs or x-rays cannot "see" the source of a problem.

Although a traumatic incident may seem like ancient history, your body remembers the trauma long after the mental memory fades. One example the physiatrist gives is piriformis syndrome, in which discomfort is almost always isolated to one leg. Yet in the lab, researchers have found no anatomical differences between the right and left buttocks, which indicates a functional cause.

Pain can come and go. Yet it's all too common for the irritations to play hide-and-seek when you finally get to the doctor's office, which can make it a bit more challenging for your healthcare professional.

The list of conditions that cause pain is extensive. For example:

- More than half of pregnant women can have back pain at some point.
- Both sciatica and sacroiliac (SI) joint derangement can flare up as the mother-to-be's body changes.
- Spinal stenosis and osteoarthritis are more common with age.
- Herniated and slipped discs are often associated with athletes and overuse.
- Rheumatoid arthritis is an autoimmune disease that can occur at any age.

A multitude of specialists, like Dr. Fishman, exists because there is such a broad range of potential issues.

When it comes to the back, there are primarily two types of pain:

1. Nerve (or neurological) pain is induced by issues like spinal stenosis or a herniated disc.
2. Structural (or musculoskeletal) pain has its origin in conditions like SI joint derangement.

Some sources of pain are both neurological and structural, such as piriformis syndrome, where structure (muscle) interferes with the sciatic nerve. Arthritis pain can also result from either structural or neurological causes.

In the end, according to Dr. Fishman, 80 percent of back pain is musculoskeletal. This suggests that most pain is related to the mechanics of the bones and muscles.

In the past, doctors encouraged bed rest for many conditions. However, lying immobile often exacerbates pain. Many people start yoga when their backs are bothering them. That said, anyone turning to yoga for the potential benefits must alert their teacher or provider to the fact that they are experiencing pain (or other chronic issues).

Yoga is not necessarily one-size-fits-all, especially for those with neurological or musculoskeletal conditions, which is why yoga therapists traditionally perform at least a sixty-minute intake with each new client.

The doctor explains:

> Yoga is the best means I know of for reducing back pain to manageable levels, if not completely abolishing it and keeping it from becoming a dominant factor in your life. Yoga relieves pain and promotes calm to endure any pain that remains. It can address back pain generally through prevention and directly with attention to the specific cause of existing pain.

That persistent dull ache in the lower back is often caused by weak or tight muscles, which can be triggered by the common culprits of excess weight, improper posture, or sedentary lifestyles.

In some cultures, people of all ages sit on the ground and squat. In the West, we sink into large, soft chairs or couches. Marketing and society say the softer the better; yet the softer it is, the worse the effects on the back. Our couch potato culture turns us into The Tin Man, devoid of flexibility and muscle tone.

Fortunately, yoga is accessible to everyone. Plus, Dr. Fishman asserts while cracking a smile, you don't have to spend hours sweating to get a positive effect.

> Yoga does unusual things to the bones. It pulls them in uncommon ways. Yoga is better than weight lifting since groups of muscles, each stronger than gravity, oppose one another in *asana* (yoga postures). We can generate forces far more than what gravity can. Well, maybe not on Jupiter.

Asana builds bone density and strength. In addition, the venerable practice improves coordination, range of motion, balance and mental alertness, which can help to prevent trips or falls. A great thing about yoga is that it is relatively easy and adaptable for everyone. Pregnant women, the elderly and amputees can all benefit from an adaptable yoga practice.

What makes the prescription of yoga even more inviting is that, in as little as ten minutes a day, you can keep the doctor away.

> Yoga and arthritis were made for each other. The hallmark of arthritis is lack of range of motion. If yoga does anything, it stretches, which increases range of motion.

There are more than one hundred types of arthritis, a leading cause of disability in the United States, which affects more than fifty million adults and three hundred thousand children. The first line of defense is movement, since inactivity exacerbates the condition. While any form of movement therapy is beneficial, yoga has an arsenal of bonuses.

Consider bone spurs, which can appear at any age. Those stony jagged projections can inhibit range of motion. With the growth of bone spurs in the spine, for example, the disc spacing can narrow and, if there is insufficient lubrication, bending or arching of the back can be uncomfortable. While it may seem counterintuitive to move when it hurts, with yoga, there are substantial benefits, especially for those with bone spurs.

> There is evidence that practicing yoga can actually improve the smoothness and symmetry of the two surfaces of a joint. Yoga appears to work to realign the underlying rows of cells that produce the joint surface collagen. It could be that a joint will never return to the condition it was in when you were two years old, but yoga will definitely help.

Then there are the positive emotional and spiritual side effects of practicing yoga. While some in the medical community will not mention it, these side effects contribute to the healing process. Yoga, plain and simple, makes you feel good.

Dr. Fishman effusively notes:

> [There is] the pleasure of doing yoga. If you want to do yoga right, do it every day—including Sundays and bank holidays.

Dr. Fishman's Five Easy Tips

1. Get a diagnosis from a qualified professional before starting anything.
   Many people prefer multiple opinions from different specialists. Then, follow an individual treatment plan from a qualified yoga therapist or other specialist who is experienced in your condition.

Don't just follow a video tutorial or group class without first discussing with a specialist which yoga poses can soothe or aggravate the pain, depending on the issue.

2. **Find relief from herniated discs.**
Usually, the pain of herniated discs can be eased with backbending yoga poses, like sphinx,[73] fish[74] or bridge,[75] with or without supports. It is essential to know to which side the disc is protruding before attempting any particular yoga position.

3. **Soothe dull lower backaches.**
For those whose diagnosis confirms no neurological issues, building core strength is helpful. Too often people strain their back when their abdominal and limb muscles are not doing the work. Planks[76] and sun salutations[77] can help by building core support to counteract the back muscles overexerting themselves. While each yoga lineage may have a different variation, sun salutations incorporate gentle backbends and forward folds, partial inversions with downward dogs, and *dorsiflexion* (pulling the top of the foot in an upward direction toward the body) and *plantar flexion* (flexing the foot or toes downward toward the sole).

4. **Address piriformis syndrome.**
When piriformis syndrome is causing problems, it can be offset by opening the spaces between the piriformis muscle in the buttocks and the sciatic nerve on the offending side. The best exercises are deep twists where you can feel the stretch in the sensitive area. Suggested yoga poses, provided there

are no other spinal injuries, include half lord of the
fishes[78] and the twisted triangle.[79]

5. Counteract the effects of spondylolisthesis.
Often caused by a sports injury, this occurs when
one vertebra slides (usually forward) onto the one
beneath it. Stretching and strengthening the lower
back is often beneficial. The boat pose[80] is a yoga
exercise that can be adapted based on your existing
core strength. Depending on your abilities, different
positions may be suggested to increase or decrease
the difficulty of the asana. As with herniations, get
an official diagnosis and green light from your doctor
before engaging in any exercise.

Backing Up Yoga for Back Pain

I can personally affirm the benefits of yoga for back pain. I
first experienced sharp, lumbar pain as an adolescent. My
lower back would spasm when getting into or out of a chair.
Imaging identified a minor congenital deviation at the coccyx.
The orthopedist I was seeing guided me in exercises to flatten
out the excessive curvature in my spine and strengthen my
abdominal muscles.

That was how I first began practicing the physical components of yoga—in response to almost unbearable pain. While
I have not felt that agony since I was a teen, I still (try to) limber
up my back and strengthen my core daily. Any periodic dull
aches are easily silenced with a relaxed position, bending
forward at the waist, like a rag doll[81] and child's pose.[82] If I sit
in a chair or couch, tension creeps into my lower back. On
the other hand, I can sit erect on the floor for hours comfortably. Leaning against a wall or chair back is a no-no for me. I

learned long ago that type of positioning is a problem for my structural health.

In more recent diagnoses, they found bone spurs and arthritis in my hands and shoulders. Even though these conditions exist, I have an exceptional range of motion and zero pain. Just as I recognize my blood sugar would be through the roof if I followed the Standard American Diet and lifestyle, I don't doubt I would have discomfort and stiffness if I were a couch potato. I keep my body and joints moving throughout the day, and sometimes in the middle of the night, to avoid issues that being more static would promote. When not performing sun salutations or yoga poses, I do targeted exercises, like joint rotations. I am conscious of opportunities to keep in motion in the car, in bed and even in the bathtub.

While I am convinced that yoga helped my back pain and am impressed by Dr. Fishman's abundance of work, there are independent studies to back up my conclusion.

Yoga, tai chi and qi gong were the focus of a Chinese systematic review and meta-analysis published in 2019.[83] The study confirmed that each of the mindful practices reduced chronic lower back pain.

In Switzerland, three researchers at the University of Geneva's Institute of Global Health assessed Iyengar yoga to reduce back pain.[84] They concluded that "The practice of yoga can decrease pain and increase functional ability in patients with spinal pain."

A medical school in Turkey compared isometrics, yoga and Pilates for chronic neck pain. Measures of success ranged from the alleviation of pain to increased quality of life and improved emotional state. After six weeks of treatment, all three groups experienced a decrease in pain, with a side effect of better moods.

Stateside, a military medical center led a randomized control trial among people with chronic lower back pain. The conclusion: eight weeks of yoga was a viable treatment option with minimal side effects.[85]

Dr. Khalsa (who you met in "Chapter 2: Yoga as an Emotional Lifesaver") spearheaded a study on lower back pain in conjunction with a Boston teaching hospital. After eight weeks, there were drastic reductions in all measures of pain using a common self-administered measure of disability. In addition, levels of perceived stress, depression and fatigue dropped.

There is plenty of documentation that proves the effectiveness of yoga postures to minimize back pain. When diagnosed and then guided by qualified professionals, yoga is an enjoyable form of therapy that costs a fraction of what traditional treatments can run, entails no recuperation periods, and has no negative side effects or risks of potentially fatal addictions.

Give It a Try:
Warm Up the Spine

The following six-directional exercise[86] lubricates and limbers a healthy spine per the natural anatomical movement patterns: forward, backward, left, right, twist left and twist right.

For those with pre-existing conditions, as always, ask your healthcare provider before starting. A few contraindications are noted below. As a rule of thumb, don't do anything that causes pain or discomfort.

1. **Get comfortable.**

   Come to a seated position on the floor or, if preferred, on a hard chair. Sit tall. Reach the crown of your head to the sky. Relax. Inhale and exhale through the nose.

Then, place each palm on the corresponding knee or wherever you feel you can grasp, such as the base of your chair or your thigh.

2. **Do the seated cat/cow.**

For the first two directions, inhale and arch your torso backward, opening up the chest and lungs, then exhale and round forward as if someone is punching you in the stomach, unless you have osteoporosis. If you don't have cervical spine issues, move your head in conjunction with your spine, lifting your chin with the arching and bowing your head with the rounding. Repeat for a minute, ensuring that each movement flows slowly with your breathing.

3. **Perform lateral side stretches.**

This exercise can be done with the hands and arms in many positions. In this version, place your right fingertips on the floor (or chair) next to you as you reach your left hand and fingers high to the sky. Breathe deeply, lengthening your spine. As you exhale, let your right elbow bend and reach the left arm up and over your head. Leading with your right shoulder, allow the upper torso to sink to the right. Take several deep breaths. With each inhalation, feel the spaces between your left ribs expand. After about twenty seconds, repeat in the other direction.

4. **Twist your torso.**

Note: This step is not appropriate for pregnant women or people with spinal fusions.

Again, there are many variations to this movement. The following is a traditional kundalini yoga twist. Place your hands on their respective shoulders with your thumbs behind and the rest of your fingers in front of your shoulder while pointing your elbows to the side. Inhale as you twist left; exhale, twisting right. Find a rhythm that works best for your breath. Keep your head in alignment with the spine, unless you have cervical spine issues or are prone to dizziness. Repeat for about a minute.

5. Rest.

   When done, stay still and notice how your entire body, breath and mind feel.

Now it's time to turn over and focus on the belly rather than the back.

Chapter 6: Go with Your Gut

I believe in nature's cures.

—Dr. P. R. Vishnu

The life science of Ayurveda originated in India and dates back several thousand years. Like traditional Chinese medicine, it is widely accepted as a complete health system and modern science has confirmed its efficacy. Unlike Western healthcare, Ayurveda is prevention-focused and strives to identify the root causes of disease. This chapter reveals why almost all health issues can be traced to what you put in your mouth and your belly's reaction to it.

After I completed my yoga teacher training, I went to India to study Ayurveda, yoga's sister science. I chose a program at a Sivananda ashram in a rainforest in Kerala, the Ayurvedic world capital.

While it was an introductory course, it was tough. P. R. Vishnu, BAMS, MD, was our lead teacher. He drummed data into our heads using analogies and stories. He often approached his lessons with flashing eyes and a hearty laugh; a toothy smile peeking out from under his mustache.

Lectures and practice sessions were Mondays through Saturdays. One Sunday, there was a perk: an outing to an Ayurvedic hospital, pharmacy and botanical farm. Afterward, we went sightseeing to Kanyakumari, where three bodies of water unite at the southernmost tip of India.

Although we were playing tourists, this day was an Ayurvedic crash course too. We learned how to sniff out the three body and mind constitution *doshas*[87] of *vata*,[88] *pitta*,[89] and *kapha*[90] with simple observations. It is a practice that can take years to master.

One of our impromptu exercises was at a small roadside diner. Everyone was served the same dish, with our choice of Indian bread. Seeing the clueless expressions of the Westerners in our group, Dr. Vishnu placed the orders based on our doshic imbalances. He gave me a quick visual once-over, identified my dosha, and said, "You get the poori."

After lunch, waiting to board a ferry along with a few hundred others, we asked how he assessed our constitution without the tried-and-true pulse test and thorough exam. There began exercise number two, learning how to detect one's dosha from characteristics and habits.

Dr. Vishnu and his associate pointed to people willy-nilly. "That person kicking his feet? That's a vata trait. The man with sweat stains on his shirt? Pitta. The young boy with darting eyes? A sign of vitiated vata," Dr. Vishnu told us.

In a matter of ten minutes, they did quick reads on upward of thirty people. It was mind-blowing to watch the masters pinpoint subtle qualities manifested in the constitutions. In our society, we tend to focus on styles, shapes and colors of one's wardrobe, accessories, hair and skin. But the Ayurvedic practitioner sees the person's behavior along with those traits that manifest in physical characteristics, such as reddish complexion or long curly eyelashes.

Dr. Vishnu taught us that even body odors correlate to one's elemental constitution. Highlighting the importance of gut health, he told us that Indian parents check on their kids' bowel movements every morning. If there is no activity, they provide a natural remedy. The size, shape and frequency of what goes into the toilet is a key to reading one's doshic balance or imbalance.

The Doctor in the Dining Hall: Dr. P. R. Vishnu

As director of the Sivananda Institute of Health, Dr. Vishnu is the lead instructor of Ayurvedic studies in three countries: India, Canada and Japan. Through his Ayurvedic medical studies, he specialized in the treatment of neurological, rheumatic and bone degenerative diseases. His advanced degree is in *panchakarma*, which is the Ayurvedic approach to eliminate toxins from disease, food or the environment that bog down the body. Ayurveda is in Dr. Vishnu's blood since he comes from a family of Ayurvedic doctors.

While the 5,000-year-old life science is not common in the West, 40 to 50 percent of healthcare in Kerala is Ayurvedic. Throughout India, the plethora of Ayurvedic products, from nutraceuticals to toothpaste, generated more than $7.5 billion in sales in 2022.[91]

From the time Vishnu was a child, he had a passion to learn more about herbal and natural remedies.

> Many people are unaware that Ayurveda is based on living principles that can treat many chronic disorders by lifestyle changes. Ayurveda is extremely beneficial, and I wanted to use this life

science to help people. I believe in nature's cures
and healthy lifestyles.

The ancient preventive and curative holistic approach to opti-
mizing one's health is divided into eight branches: general
medicine; pediatrics and obstetrics/gynecology; surgery;
ear, nose and throat; toxicology; rejuvenation; aphrodisiacs;
and psychiatry.

The energetic doctor wears many hats. Given the importance of karma yoga, or selfless service, in the Sivananda tradition, Dr. Vishnu runs a free clinic. Each month, his team of
twelve treats one thousand disadvantaged villagers.

Besides Ayurvedic training sessions like the one I attended,
he guides more than three hundred students every year in the
intricacies of the cleansing specialty of panchakarma. During
the hot summer months, he travels far beyond Kerala, heading
to Sivananda ashrams near Quebec and Tokyo, where he
works as both an instructor and clinician.

The Guru's Wisdom: Feed Your Constitution

Among the many advantages of Ayurveda is that it is all-nat-
ural, has no harmful side effects, strengthens the immune
system, and wards off disease.

Individuality is not the crux of Western medicine. Western
doctors often tap into handheld devices for diagnoses and
treatments. In contrast, the Indian wellness system recognizes that you are unique. While allopathic medicine is too
often antidote-based, the philosophy, therapy and system of
Ayurveda focuses on the underlying imbalances.

Good-intentioned Western doctors often complain about
the system of "treat and street," where clinics push patients
in and out of offices like a revolving door. Because Ayurveda
is patient-centric and not pill-focused, consultations are thor-

ough. Questions not on the radar to most allopathic doctors are routine for the Ayurvedic practitioner. For example, elimination, sleep, dreams, cravings and temper are part of an Ayurvedic consult. Without ignoring traditional lab results, Ayurvedic doctors have their own evaluation tools. While they examine your eyes, tongue and skin, they also test multiple pulse points on both wrists, not unlike traditional Chinese medicine practitioners.

According to Dr. Vishnu:

> Ayurveda believes that the medicine or course of treatment that works for one individual may not work for another. It all depends on their specific constitution and current pathological condition. For example, take two smokers. One might [develop] high cholesterol, and the other one might not. It depends on their individual constitution. So, we don't believe in treating symptoms. Symptoms are considered an imbalance of the internal organs or digestive system. We aim at correcting the root of the problem. Because of this, there is some degree of trial and error to see what works for each individual.

In today's fast-paced society, too often people want a quick fix. However, Band-Aids never stick forever. If your diet has been poor your entire life, one good meal does not make a difference. Ayurveda aims for the bull's eye, with narrow-focused lifestyle modifications.

The doctor adds:

> Ayurveda is a gradual system of healing. It focuses on correcting dietary discipline and making life-

style changes. At times, people are not very comfortable making these big changes.

Imagine the chronic obstructive pulmonary disease patient who will not quit smoking or the person with liver damage who keeps reaching for the beer or whiskey bottle.

> If someone has a skin disorder, steroids might be prescribed and bring temporary, immediate relief. But the issue will recur. Ayurveda treats the root of the disorder and its recurrence.

Precisely because Ayurveda is not one-size-fits-all, the Indian medical methodology can be hard to understand. The approach is not as simple and quick as taking an aspirin for your headache or an antihistamine for your runny nose. Instead, it is about balance, which results in well-being. Ayurveda goes far beyond identifying the aforementioned constitutions. Doshas alone are not enough, as they are in constant flux, like a three-way teeter-totter.

An Ayurvedic doctor understands how to recognize disharmony at every level of the body, from the bones to the blood to the muscles, including the *gunas*[92] (qualities or attributes invisible to Western medicine). Imbalances anywhere cause disease in the body and emotions.

On a macro level, what you eat or drink can soothe or cause chaos to your multilayered systems. The gut is the central processor for whatever you swallow. If that engine is well oiled, no problem. But when there are kinks and roadblocks or unnatural acceleration in your innards, the bedlam goes beyond the belly. The traffic controller, to a large extent, is the digestive fire (*agni*).

Dr. Vishnu explains:

> According to Ayurveda, any imbalance in our
> system is caused by irregular agni, as well as the
> accumulation of *ama* (toxic build-up) in our body.
> Ayurveda professes that all physical and most
> mental disorders originate in the gut. Unhealthy
> eating habits are the root cause of major and
> minor imbalances and diseases.

It is not a surprise that there are so many chronically ill people
in the United States. Consider the Standard American Diet
(SAD). Too often, meals and snacks are stuck in a freezer and
shoved in a microwave or picked up at a food court or drive-
through and scarfed down while watching television or
surfing the internet. Generations ago, there were limited prepared or fast food options. Breakfast, lunch and dinner were
made from scratch with love, and the entire family enjoyed
the meal together at the kitchen table.

The modern medical community acknowledges that the
Standard American Diet has contributed to epidemic propor-
tions of high blood pressure, diabetes, stress and autoimmune
diseases. According to the Centers for Disease Control (CDC)
fact sheet "Poor Nutrition," fewer than 10 percent of American
adults and adolescents eat enough fruit and vegetables.[93] More
than 70 percent of the average American's sodium intake is a
result of not eating homemade meals.[94] A high 41.9 percent of
adults are obese,[95] and one in three American adults are predi-
abetic.[96] In a CDC infographic, we learn that six in ten people
in the United States suffer from a chronic disease with four in
ten having two or more chronic diseases.[97]

Dr. Vishnu comments:

> The modern diet is unhealthy everywhere. My experiences and observations among North American people are that there exists a vicious cycle of stress and stress-related eating patterns. That impacts the digestive system and destroys agni, which creates digestive and other irregularities. A sedentary lifestyle and high-stress levels cause toxic build-up in the body, which is the root cause of all other disorders and diseases. When the diet is wrong and combined with chronic stress, it leads to autoimmune disease and other major health conditions.

The SAD diet often labels "good food" as what's tasty and filling, even if it's loaded with preservatives, sodium and sugars. From an Ayurvedic perspective, "good" equals fresh. *Sattvic* foods are pure, fresh, nonaggravating and balancing to the gunas. Therefore, you should strive to consume more of them. On the other hand, *tamasic* foods (old, recooked or processed) may be lethargy producing or toxic and can negatively impact digestion. Eating in a hurry or without savoring the food slows digestive efficiency, leading to gastrointestinal disorders and metabolic disease.

Ayurveda recommends set mealtimes—no skipping meals and no snacking or bingeing. Our digestive fire, the ability to process and absorb nutrients, is strongest from 10 a.m. to 2 p.m. The heaviest meal of the day should be during those hours.

Stressful schedules infringe on slow-paced midday family meal routines that were once common practice. People work late, come home stressed, and pop dinner into the microwave or call for pizza delivery. With time at a premium, people don't even sit and chew their food. When food is gobbled down, your intestines have to work overtime. Digestion begins with chewing, when enzymes in the saliva play their part in the digestive process. All these modern, mindless habits are the perfect storm for wreaking havoc on the digestive system.

While it may sound as if we need a total lifestyle about-face, simple dietary changes can make a big difference in our digestive well-being. Consulting an Ayurvedic doctor is the best bet for that total recharge. But at the very least, take the reins in your own hands and switch off or turn down disease-causing habits.

The Ayurvedic mantra is to eat according to your constitution. Understand the effects of the different seasons and parts of the day, some of which are intuitive. For example, ice cream or frozen yogurt are fine on a hot summer day, but not on a cold, damp evening. Bananas and pineapple are tasty in the tropics, but these fruits are not meant to be shipped across the globe to locales where they never grow. There are many reasons for the trend to seek locally grown foods or farm-to-table dining, but Ayurveda's principles are to eat locally and seasonally for better digestion, fewer allergic reactions, and balanced doshas.

Another Ayurvedic concept is to incorporate flavors that are best suited for doshic balance. We are not talking chocolate or vanilla. Ayurveda assigns all foods and spices to one of six "flavors:" salty, sweet, sour, bitter, astringent and pungent. Those need to be balanced depending on one's constitution. For example, kaphas do best with bitter, pungent and astringent vegan foods, whereas the pitta-dominant person should avoid salty, sour and spicy foods.

Dr. Vishnu explains:

> People must be aware of their individual dosha and restrict their intake of acidic, sour, heavily spiced, preserved or deep-fried foods.
>
> One of our patients suffered morning body stiffness and pain in the ankle and heels. We recommended some dietary changes, like avoiding sour and acidic foods. Within a week, her stiffness and inflammation reduced significantly. This is because, according to Ayurveda, early morning pains are related to ama and acidic foods increase ama.

The Ayurvedic approach differs greatly from Western health and diet concepts. When you understand that the harmful ama is the byproduct of impaired metabolism or undigested food, it makes sense that the body is not receiving or metabolizing the proper nutrients, nor is the body expelling toxins.

To reduce the acidic content of food and drink, opt for fresh plant-based foods whenever possible and avoid coffee, sodas and alcohol. These guidelines are part of following a pure and balanced sattvic diet, which avoids meat, alcohol and other mood-enhancing substances.

Nowadays, intermittent fasting is in vogue. Ayurveda has favored periods of abstinence for thousands of years. Dr. Vishnu notes, "A liquid fast once a week helps cleanse and restore balance to the digestive system."

Skip the fancy smoothies with protein powder, in favor of fresh fruit and vegetable juices, clear soups and broths. Whatever your food choices and habits, avoid drinking anything cold and never use ice cubes. Warm water stimulates digestion and aids in the breakdown of toxins.

Dr. Vishnu's Five Easy Tips

1. **Don't eat at night.**

   Maintain at least a three-hour window between your last meal and bedtime to help digestion and sleep. As Ayurvedic wisdom teaches us, "Our body channels are closing after sunset, just like a lotus."

2. **Drink warm water.**

   To aid digestion, drink water thirty minutes before or after food, rather than during the meal. Because ginger is an excellent digestive aid, add fresh diced or sliced ginger to a pot of boiling water for homemade ginger tea.

3. **Eat homemade wholesome dishes as much as possible.**

   Avoid precooked and reheated foods that disturb the body's pH balance.

4. **Restrict or skip fermented foods, such as pickles, vinegar, tamari and alcohol.**

   These tamasic foods interfere with digestion, alertness and energy.

5. **Minimize external stressors.**

   Practice pranayama breathwork and yoga to counteract stress and stimulate physical and mental balance.

The Wisdom of the Sages

I've been aware of my stomach most of my life. As an adolescent (a common age for imbalances to present), a gastroenterologist said my chronic belly woes and periodic intense painful episodes were stress-related. Rather than suggest medications, he told me to log my diet and flare-ups.

Since then, deep breathing, meditation, herbal teas and Ayurveda have been my best friends. Beyond my self-prescribed Ayurvedic routine, I heed everything my Ayurvedic doctor says. At each consult, he adds more diet and lifestyle suggestions to my plate. In the last twenty years, my only reliving of the unbearable cramping was the morning of my father's funeral, when my body was mourning.

Dr. Vishnu's emphasis on gut health was pivotal in my evolving vocation. After completing my studies of Ayurvedic foundations at the Sivananda center, I delved deeper into the connections between digestion and ailments of body and mind. I decided to study yoga therapy with a specialization in digestive fire disorders because I identified with problems burning, simmering or stagnant in the gut.

I am not a rare bird. A 2020 epidemiological survey of seventy-three thousand adults around the globe estimated that more than 40 percent of people worldwide suffer from functional gastrointestinal disorders, also referred to as disorders of the gut-brain interaction.[98]

There are reams of research findings, many of which correlate to digestive health. Three volumes of *Pharmacognosy of Indigenous Drugs* log key nutraceutical studies, while the Ayurvedic research database of India's Central Council for Research in Ayurvedic Studies features nearly thirty thousand published research articles and abstracts.

The *Charaka Samhita* is the Ayurvedic bible. The Sanskrit word *samhita* means "collection," and Acharya Charaka is the scholar who wrote this legendary medical text. One of the tenets of his book is that as long as agni is normal, man can have a healthy and long life. Loss of agni leads to loss of life.

P. S. Byadgi, PhD, is a researcher and assistant professor at Banaras Hindu University in Varanasi, India. In a review article for the *International Journal of Research in Ayurveda and Pharmacy*, he validates the wisdom of the sage Charaka. He notes that a healthy body is reliant on agni, which is the engine for physical and emotional health. It can be managed through proper diet and lifestyle habits.[99]

Until recently, few heeded the words attributed to Hippocrates, the father of modern medicine, in which he is believed to have said "All disease begins in the gut." One of the latest trends in health management is understanding the importance of the gut microbiome. Millions of microbes from parasites to fungi, in and on the body, are key to many aspects of our physical and emotional health. The gut microbiome carries twenty-two million bacterial genes.[100]

Dr. Joseph Weiss, a gastroenterologist and medical professor at the University of California San Diego is a gut-brain microbiome dynamics expert. In a virtual lecture I attended, he said:

> The digestive track is astounding. The human brain is in constant and direct communication with the gut-brain. [Understanding the relevance of the gut microbiome] is a revolutionary change in medicine—since 95 percent of the human immune system is localized to the gut. Every illness is found to originate in the gut. Things you would have thought have nothing to do with the gut microbiome are now thought to be intimately involved [including] Parkinson's, Alzheimer's, autism, cardiovascular disease, cancers, arthritis. The list goes on and on.

Dr. Weiss explains that the gut produces hormones like tryptophan, adrenaline and norepinephrine, so it is not surprising that the twenty-two million genes of the gut microbiome affect mental health too.

Clinical psychologist and Ayurvedic practitioner Eliot Steer conducted a study on major depressive disorder and gut dysregulation that supports Ayurvedic theories. The *Journal of Ayurveda and Integrative Medicine* published his report in 2019, in which he states:

> There are some striking similarities between this biomedical understanding of the gastrointestinal system and the Ayurvedic perspective of disease development... Both Ayurveda and current approaches in biomedicine seek to understand the causation of depression as it relates to the gastrointestinal system, as well as identifying treatment modalities that specifically target this link.[101]

Acknowledging the connection between emotions and digestive fire, Steer notes improper diet can cause imbalances, leading to insomnia and what he calls "disturbed thoughts."

> More than thirty different neurotransmitters are used by the gut in regulating functioning and in communication with the brain via the vagus nerve.

According to Steer, personalized Ayurvedic treatment of major depressive disorder can be more effective than the allopathic standards of care and lead patients to longer-lasting positive outcomes.

To sum it up, when you focus on your digestive health, you address both physical and emotional well-being.

Give It a Try:
Do-It-Yourself Tea

A tea made from cumin, coriander and fennel has calming and cleansing effects. It is inexpensive and easy to make.

Each of the ingredients helps with digestion. Together, they are more potent and balance the doshas. The combination is also said to boost the absorption of nutrients and cleanse the lymphatic system.

Preparation time: five minutes.

1. Take equal amounts of cumin, coriander and fennel seeds.

2. Mix and store in an empty spice container or similar small bottle.

3. Add about ¼ teaspoon of the combined seeds to 2 cups of water.

4. Boil and let steep for at least 5 minutes.

5. Strain, sip, relax and enjoy the herbal potion. It is not sweet or spicy, so you may want to add a drop or two of agave.

Now that you have a basic understanding of Ayurveda and sattvic diets, we will explore the benefits of a sattvic lifestyle.

Chapter 7: Your Choices Matter

*Animals sometimes behave
in a much more rational way than humans do.*

—Chaitanya Charan Das

On my second trip to India, I expected quality time with His Holiness Radhanath Swami. (You'll read more about him in "Chapter 11: Happiness Isn't a Big Bank Account.") Just a few days before our departure, the leaders revised the itinerary, adding daily lectures by two Indian monks. My reaction was not positive since listening to long speeches puts me to sleep.

My worries were for naught. The presence of these shaven-headed men dressed in orange robes was the highlight of the trip for me. During our journey through northern India, our last-minute add-on monks spoke about engaging topics from love to man versus ape. They selected sacred relics and historic monuments for our open-air lecture halls.

One unforgettable class was held on a hilltop, an image of which graces the cover of one of Radhanath Swami's autobiographies. The holy site was a picture-perfect, sunny, breezy, peaceful place, except for the infamous packs of small monkeys known for stealing the eyeglasses and hats of visitors. While the monks led us, a nearby guard was responsible for shooing the monkeys away.

With our attention focused on the monks, their lesson's takeaway was that there are many ways to get to the top of a hill. Many prefer slower zigzagging or circular routes. Others sprint to the summit, whereas some may take breaks along the way. No one path is the right way. The monks used the way up the hill as an analogy for spirituality. It does not matter which approach or religion you follow. All roads lead toward the same God, regardless of the name you assign it.

Our monks were level-headed, interesting, intelligent and well-spoken teachers who fit in well with our tight-knit and religiously diverse group. Their presence amounted to having personal gurus on our domestic plane trips, slow-moving bus journeys, bumpy rickshaw rides, and long walks.

One of the two monks, Chaitanya Charan Das, gave up his software engineer attire in favor of a saffron-colored robe. This Vaishnava monk is a prolific author, lecturer, podcaster, video host, editor and blogger who takes an analytical approach to extol the virtues of a plant-based, drug-free lifestyle.

Chaitanya, also known as the "spiritual scientist," may be a renunciate, who opted for simplicity, celibacy and detachment, but he is plugged into worldwide current events, public opinion, and modern technology. His rational discussions and questions steered me to better understand simple things in life that often go unexplored. I appreciated how Chaitanya approached all issues with respect for diverse practices and peoples.

Upon my return to the States, I read Chaitanya's books, followed him on social media, and connected with him through virtual lectures. Even as he was on the other side of the globe, he fueled my brain and soul. His discussions were far from boring. So much so that I rejoined both monks in India for three weeks in 2023. The wide range of matters Chaitanya analyzed from a historic and cultural vantage point included marriages, the caste system, and sattvic (vegetarian and drug-free) lifestyles. The last topic hit a chord.

Our traveling guru's understanding of human nature gave me more clarity. It reinforced and rationalized my long-standing instincts while helping me to be less judgmental.

A plethora of websites and books exist touting meat-free meals. Even more prevalent are the awareness and agreement surrounding the injurious effects of smoking, excessive drinking and taking recreational drugs. Most discussion focuses on the physical detriments. Yet there are emotional and spiritual side effects to what we choose to consume as well.

The Spiritual Scientist: Chaitanya Charan Das

Chaitanya Charan's life experiences taught him to listen to his instincts. He felt compelled to choose the road less traveled. He eschewed a traditional life.

Born Chandrahas Pujari, his first name means "laugh like the moon" in Hindi, and his surname refers to a priest. At about the time that most tots begin to walk, Chandrahas' legs couldn't hold up his tiny body. Concerned, his mother and father took him to the doctor, who gave a grim diagnosis. A defective polio vaccine had never protected the toddler. He had contracted polio and would never be able to walk unaided.

Before he turned four, little Chandrahas faced two serious injuries. The first was from a firecracker explosion. All the other kids ran away. He could not. Second- and third-degree burns covered his arm and face. Not long after that, he had a frightening fall, resulting in a fractured skull.

His parents did a good job of keeping his spirits high. While he may not have kept up with the kids on the sports field, he surpassed them all in the classroom. His fascination for research and observation led him to excel at school from his early years until he graduated from college at the top of his class.

> I felt that the scientific spirit of inquiry could offer intelligent answers to the questions of the inquisitive mind. Also, that technology—television, cars, airplanes and computers—would make India modern and progressive.

That inquisitive mind didn't allow him to take a back seat. It disheartened and perplexed him as he watched two of his brilliant colleagues make foolish and ultimately fatal decisions.

As Chandrahas faced a personal crossroads, he pondered those two deaths. He was the first student at the University of Pune, in the West Indian state of Maharashtra, to earn a near-perfect score on the Graduate Record Examinations. He received invitations from first-rate graduate schools in the United States, yet he turned down the opportunity to study abroad. Instead, he chose to stay in India and immerse himself in spirituality and the yoga of devotion, bhakti.

> There were many who would be more than happy to take my seat in an American science college. There were very few who would become scientific spokespersons for bhakti yoga.

Distressed by the effects of the addictive behaviors of those close to him, he found answers in the *Bhagavad Gita*, the ancient "Song of the Lord." He embraced the logical discussions among the devotees of the International Society for Krishna Consciousness (ISKCON).

While talking about his decision to follow the nonmaterial path, he shared:

> The struggle to reconcile the lofty ideals I cherished with the lousy reality I observed around me prompted me to turn to spirituality for answers. It was *because* of my scientific propensity, not despite it. My scientific instincts made me look at spirituality with a healthy dose of skepticism.

In 1999, Chandrahas deepened his commitment to bhakti. He found his greatest teacher, Radhanath Swami, who gave him the spiritual name Chaitanya Charan Das when he opted to renounce materialism and married life to become a monk. The Sanskrit word *chaitanya* means "spirit" or "intelligence." *Charan* denotes moral conduct and *das* stands for "servant (of the Lord)."

Many years later, his faith was put to the test while practicing his morning japa mantra meditation. He was at one of ISKCON's temples in Mumbai, focused on repeating the names of the Lord while fingering his prayer beads. Unaware of a puddle of water on the marble floor, he slipped. The brace supporting his paralytic leg caused an unnatural torque at the upper thigh. As a result, the fall caused a severe break in and dislocation of an osteoporotic femur.

> Not only was the [physical] pain unbearable, but it was a faith crisis. I was absorbed in the mood of prayer, in a temple of God, chanting the names of God. Why didn't the divine protect me?

Amid excruciating pain, he focused on holy *sutras* (threads or lines that offer spiritual teachings) for several hours before surgery.

> The *Bhagavad Gita* has seven hundred verses, and I have memorized most of them. As soon as I started reciting them, I found my pain almost mystically disappearing. If for one moment I stopped, even to catch my breath, the pain returned.

The radiologist and the emergency room doctor were stunned at Chaitanya's state of calm. They had to verify that the x-rays were his. He recalls:

> That experience was both physically and spiritually challenging. Transcending the pain was almost magical. It deepened my faith. Through sonic meditation, we can create a buffer between ourselves and our troubles.

The Guru's Wisdom: Think Before You Eat

For many of us, eating and drinking are habitual acts. Are you really starving when you eat that bag of potato chips? Is your body really dehydrated when you gulp down a supersized soda? Chaitanya encourages people to stop, ponder and reevaluate their habits of consumption and opt for a pure and balanced diet.

Fifty years ago, it was challenging for Westerners with dietary restrictions to find nourishment. Nowadays, despite the abundance of junk foods, nourishing options are much more accessible, regardless of your chosen diet.

To begin with, if you assess the human body versus that of other species, it is clear we are not meant to feast on other animals. Most primates are herbivores. Chimpanzees, our closest kin, share 99 percent of our DNA. Like us, they are capable of eating and digesting meat. While most monkeys are vegetarians, Jane Goodall observed chimps eating insects back in the 1960s. This was less the norm than a rare delicacy. According to the Goodall Institute, animal products account for a mere 6 percent of the great ape's diet.

Chaitanya clarifies that although our bodies can process animal flesh, we are not made for meat consumption. This seems to be confirmed by our anatomy. The hands, fingers, mouth, jaw, teeth, intestines, colon and even pH balance in our digestive tract do not reflect the characteristics of strict carnivores.

> Mother Nature could hardly have made a clearer statement about what sort of diet is natural for humans than what she has already done through the features of human anatomy. From the small number of canine teeth to the relatively longer intestine, which characterizes herbivores, our body is more suited for an herbivorous diet, and therefore, a plant-based diet is healthier.

Many medical practitioners, especially cardiologists, agree. Eating meat does not do our body good. Nor is it kind to the planet.

Chaitanya offers the acronym HELP to outline his rationale for why your choices can have a positive impact on our health, environment, livestock and poverty.[102]

H = Improve Your Health

Most vegans[103] hear a constant barrage of questions from meat-eaters asking how they get enough protein. Yet herbivorous elephants, rhinoceros and hippopotami are among the largest and strongest in the animal kingdom. Many star athletes and even bodybuilders choose plant-based diets. So it is a misconception that we need to bulk up on beef for strength.

In his article, Chaitanya refers to statements from the Physicians Committee for Responsible Medicine, a nonprofit organization based in Washington, DC, composed of seventeen thousand physicians around the world. Their fact sheet "The Protein Myth" cautions against high-protein diets.[104]

The average American consumes about double the protein their body needs.[105] In addition, the primary sources of protein consumed tend to be animal products, which are also high in unhealthy fats. It surprises most individuals to learn that protein needs are actually much less than what they have been consuming.

The Physicians Committee website provides more glaring evidence.

> Protein deficiency is almost unheard of in the United States. It's easy to get all the protein you need without eating meat, dairy or eggs... More isn't always better. One study found that people eating large amounts of animal protein have twenty-three times the risk of death from diabetes and five times the risk of death from cancer as those consuming less protein.

A meat-centered diet contributes to osteoporosis, cancer, heart disease and impaired kidney functioning.

E = Defend the Environment

The meat industry is a major contributor to climate change and loss of biodiversity. The massive ranches and slaughterhouses spew out destructive methane, nitrous oxide and carbon dioxide emissions. That was why Sir Paul McCartney has long supported the Meat Free Monday campaign with the slogan "One day a week can make a world of difference."

Chaitanya writes:

> Meat eating also has hazardous effects on the environment, such as forest destruction, agricultural inefficiency, soil erosion and desertification, air pollution, water depletion, and water pollution.
>
> The environmental fallouts of assembly-line meat factories don't end with water and air pollution. They extend far beyond to include enormous amounts of energy and the consumption of ever-increasing amounts of grain, which also leads to staggering deforestation.

To illustrate the point, Chaitanya refers to a Japanese study that equated carbon dioxide emissions from the production of just 2.2 pounds of beef to that of a European car driving more than 155 miles.[106]

L = Protect Our Livestock

The factory farming industry is brutal. Watch any behind-the-scenes video and it will make you rethink eating a chicken nugget, hot dog, sausage link or even grilled cheese or scrambled eggs. Today's largest food suppliers are not your small-time Old MacDonald or Farmer in the Dell, whose barn is a stone's throw from the owner's house and whose pastures double as the children's playground.

Chances are, your ancestors had a few farm animals to provide extra food for the family. Although there is a trend to return to growing your own pesticide-free plants and having a chicken coop in your backyard, the vast majority of food products are from enormous factory farms. While small or independent farms account for 20 percent of all food produced today, they only provide for 1 percent of the meat, dairy and eggs eaten in the United States. Due to squelching competition from large corporate farming operations, much of the food produced by smaller farms aren't sold to the average consumer. Instead, they're bought by factory farms as animal feed or by corporations for ethanol.

To maximize profits for factory farms, dairy cows are artificially impregnated every year. Their calves are inhumanely forced away from the mother after just a day or two, whereas the natural cycle for a calf is nine months of suckling and a lifetime alongside its mother. Once the offspring are separated, the males, seen as profitable tender veal cuts, are confined in tight crates to prevent them from building muscle. The females are isolated and impregnated earlier than normal to continue the production cycle.

In contrast, Chaitanya's spiritual organization runs small dairy farms from Italy to India that follow the motto "Do no harm." Since their beloved cows are treated tenderly rather than with only profitability in mind, the organic dairy output is limited and considered a treat. The residents and guests often savor traditional Indian-style desserts made from their sacred cows' milk.

Nonviolent farming is rare, as Chaitanya notes:

> Hens are so tightly packed in battery cages that they cannot move an inch. Constantly rubbing against the wire cages, they suffer from severe feather loss, and their bodies are covered with bruises and abrasions. They are forced by chemical manipulation to lay about 200–220 eggs every

year, leading to weakened bones and several other painful maladies.

If you saw the 2020 movie *Minari*, about Korean immigrants working on a chicken farm in Arkansas, you know the female chickens are the lucky ones.

According to Chaitanya:

> Because male chicks can't lay eggs, they are of no economic value. They are ruthlessly disposed of by being tossed into trash cans or plastic bags, where they undergo excruciating deaths by suffocation or by being crushed under the weight of other chicks. In some cases, they are mercilessly ground to powder (while still alive) so their remains can be made into fertilizer.

P = Stand Against Poverty

Hunger is a global issue according to the 2020 State of Food Security and Nutrition in the World annual report.[107] There are six hundred ninety million people chronically undernourished or experiencing severe food insecurity, often a result of insufficient financial resources to consume nutrient-rich food items. Another two billion have moderate-to-severe food insecurity, and one hundred thirty-five million are in a temporary crisis level of food shortage.[108]

Starvation is not just a concern in developing countries. There is a great deal of food insecurity in first-world nations too. At the height of the 2020 coronavirus epidemic, with its resulting unprecedented levels of unemployment, one in nine New Yorkers were part of the food-insecure population. Associated Press journalists Luis Andres Henao and Jessie Wardarski reported, "In New York City alone, an estimated two million residents are facing food insecurity."[109]

According to David Pimentel, professor of ecology at Cornell University's College of Agriculture and Life Sciences, more than half of cereal grains grown in the United States sustain livestock rather than humans.

> The meat-based food system requires more energy, land and water resources than the lactoovovegetarian diet. At present, the US livestock population consumes more than seven times as much grain as is consumed directly by the entire American population.[110]

The fact that so many Americans struggle to put food on their table was the impetus behind former First Lady Michelle Obama's White House Kitchen Garden. She was aware of poor nutrition that was aggravated by food deserts—locations with limited access to affordable and nutritious food because there are no supermarkets, only high-priced convenience stores that do not stock fresh fruit and vegetables. With the help of school kids, she created a food supply garden in the White House and later wrote a book, *The Story of the White House Kitchen Garden and Gardens Across America.*[111]

Feed Your Soul

The spiritual community Chaitanya belongs to, The International Society for Krishna Consciousness, discourages carnivorous diets, drinking alcohol, gambling and casual sex.

ISKCON teaches that when individuals are misguided by anger, intoxication, desire, greed and even eating meat, they can turn into a slave of these habits. For example, a toddler never chooses to kill an animal or become intoxicated. Those behaviors are acquired.

In India, it is commonplace for people to be vegetarian teetotalers. Based on the principle of not causing harm to other living things, ISKCON preaches that spiritual life culminates in the love of God, which precipitates respect for all beings as one's brothers.

Chaitanya shares:

> Spiritually, how can we have compassion for others if we kill and feast on them? All of creation are the children of God.

If you want to change your diet, you don't have to make the switch cold turkey. There are many ways to ease off the reliance on animal products. Some people choose to start by eliminating red meats or practicing meatless Mondays. Others feel comfortable as a pescatarian. What is important is to be mindful. Recognize that any effort will have a positive impact on your health, the environment and the lives of other living creatures.

Chaitanya explains:

> Many people eat meat without even thinking there is anything wrong with it. That's what they have done throughout their childhood. They never really connected meat on their plate with the living animal who is screaming and struggling and crying as he is being ruthlessly slaughtered. That means our sense of morality, of right or wrong, is often culturally conditioned. But as [people] study scriptures and as their consciousness becomes more refined, they will feel appalled at the prospect of eating meat. So conscience is the

faculty that is there within all of us. It can become a precious asset for our spiritual journey.

Yogis are taught to be grounded in nonviolence (*ahimsa*), peace and love. However, Chaitanya notes:

> One of my greatest shocks was when I encountered the yoga world in the West. I come from India, where almost everyone who seeks spiritual growth knows that cruelty-free food is an invaluable and even indispensable element of any serious path.

Given the well-traveled monk's methodical nature, he asked meat-eating Western yogis why they did not honor ahimsa.

> For many seekers, and even for the teachers, that application of ahimsa had not even crossed their mind. Or if it had, it hadn't registered deeply because many of them live in a culture where eating meat is the norm and the prevailing culture, worldview and religion often see humans as being entitled to eating animals. Many of them come to yoga for physical or cosmetic purposes—to make their body healthier and slimmer, and even sexier. Any presentation of yoga that requires abstinence from physical pleasures will be alienating. Therefore, many yoga teachers don't speak about the importance of the obvious application of ahimsa in terms of not eating meat.

Nonviolence was Rev. Dr. Martin Luther King Jr.'s credo. In keeping with the nonviolence platform, his widow, Coretta Scott King, and son, Dexter, chose to be vegetarian.

Similar to Chaitanya's opinion, Dexter King said:

> Veganism has given me a higher level of aware-
> ness and spirituality. If you're violent to yourself
> by putting things into your body that violate its
> spirit, it will be difficult not to perpetuate that
> [violence] onto someone else.

Substances that Pollute Mind, Body and Spirit

There should be no debate as to why toxic substances, including cigarettes, alcohol or drugs, are bad for the body. However,
their impact on the mind and soul is less obvious.

Chaitanya understands mood-altering substances can give
an immediate sense of lifted spirits. But any initial deceptive
pleasure is far outweighed by the longer-term negative emotional and spiritual effects.

But people are often short-sighted, as Chaitanya explains:

> The consequences of indulgence are distressing.
> Our mind is deceived. It becomes habituated to
> such an extent that we succumb to self-decep-
> tion. We don't even realize we are addicted and are
> taking in substances that are hurting and destroy-
> ing us.

Abuse of drugs negatively affects the mind and impedes spiritual growth as attention is fixated on the craving. Chaitanya
quotes Oscar Wilde on the fierceness of addictions.

> Giving up smoking is the easiest thing in the
> world. I have done it thousands of times.

Chaitanya goes on to say:

> Although some studies may suggest that alcohol
> in moderation is not a problem, the problem is

keeping it in moderation. When we get pleasure or relief by drinking, we do not realize we are slowly becoming attached to that pleasure.

Addiction to tobacco, alcohol or drugs is a perfect example of why nonattachment is a virtue in yogic philosophy. Chaitanya cautions:

Alcohol is well-known to remove, or at least lower, the inhibitions that stop us from giving in to irrational urges. While in a few cases, this lowering of inhibitions can be beneficial, the potential hazards are high.

Beyond the many accidents and fatalities caused by driving under the influence, there are endless cases of domestic violence and other acts of aggression triggered by substance abuse. Recreational drugs and alcohol mute the conscience.

Science and technology have given us access to external powers but not to internal power. Instead of simple living and high thinking, people are simply living and hardly thinking.

Without that inner power, it is harder to stop unhealthy addictions, be they smoking, drinking, gambling, taking methamphetamines or opioids, or engaging in compulsive or risky sexual behavior. While humans are supposed to be the smartest of all the animals, they don't always use their brains—or willpower—when it comes to consumption.

Many faith-based programs help people turn from unhealthy habits. The University of Michigan Addiction Research Center evaluated the connection between spirituality and recovery. Interestingly enough, religiosity did not change, but spirituality rose as individuals overcame their reliance on alcohol. Those with enhanced spirituality were more likely to remain sober.[112]

Chaitanya Charan's Five Easy Tips

1. **Remember, you are what you eat.**
   If you feed on unhealthy food, you will be unhealthy. Recognize that toxic food and drink, including those that are produced under duress or in an inhumane manner, have adverse effects on the mind, body and spirit.

2. **Appreciate wholesome vegetarian food with all the senses.**
   Take the time to enjoy the smell, taste, texture and sight of whatever you take in. As for sound, yogis often eat in silence to be more mindful of every bite.

3. **Eat at the same time every day.**
   Try to settle into a routine. Humans thrive on patterns. Eating at fixed times helps digestion and can fend off cravings.

4. **Pick healthy snacks.**
   It is best to avoid eating between meals. But if you cannot hold off until official mealtime, go with something healthy from God's garden, like apples, nuts or seeds.

5. **Be mindful of what you ingest.**
   Keep a written or mental food and beverage diary. Notice how each entry affects your energy and mood.

A Plant-Based, Drug-Free Way of Life

I wish I had met Chaitanya when I was younger. Avoiding meat, tobacco and alcohol was instinctive to me. But those choices presented ongoing battles against my culture. My religion, friends and family were not on my side, nor was the media. I was the rare bird.

From the time I could talk, my immigrant grandfather conducted solo spelling bee contests with me. His voice was raspy and faint. I never saw him smoke. In fact, he quit before I was born, but the effects didn't disappear. Emphysema took its toll. An oxygen machine stood in his bedroom. Just a few puffs on a Marlboro in elementary school were enough for me to know to stay away.

Back in the early 1970s, I went on a slaughterhouse tour. I had already been skittish about meat. After that visit, I often chose to go hungry rather than eat animal flesh.

Odd as it may sound, I worked as a bartender in two countries when I was nineteen. By the time most Americans are buying their first legal drinks, I was done with alcohol.

In the '80s, living in South America, there was one vegetarian restaurant and several small holistic shops called *tiendas de naturistas* in my city. Except within those establishments, I was viewed as an oddity.

At parties, the hosts passed cigarettes, Johnny Walker Black Label, called "Johnny *Negro*," or Anisette around on platters, like cold cuts. There was no sensitivity to secondhand smoke, and it was almost offensive to turn down a drink.

In the '90s, when it was customary to smoke in public places, I advocated for, coordinated the conversion of, and promoted the first smoke-free mall in the region. Since habits are challenging to break, some shoppers gave our security guards a hard time when they were told to extinguish their cigarettes.

I avoid anything that masks the way my body feels. Altered states are not what I am after. Half-jokingly, I tell people I don't even take aspirin, recognizing that many prescribed and over-the-counter medications are not essential.

Even legal substances aren't always good for us. Deepak Chopra says our society is addicted to silver-bullet drugs. In his book, *The Healing Self*,[113] he talks about our drug-dependent culture. According to Chopra, the average seventy-year-old takes seven prescription drugs.[114]

The CDC now recommends that medical practitioners look to holistic approaches, including yoga and acupuncture, before prescribing opioids.

My friend, Juan Steigerwald, a business and life coach, agrees with Chaitanya's points. He says we must "be the change" and respect our bodies and the planet.

> For fifteen years, I struggled with dangerously high cholesterol and relied on statin drugs and other medications that had further side effects. I was on a vicious downward cycle feeling sicker every year.
>
> In 2014, after seeing data presented by Dr. Michael Greger, an American physician and author of *How Not To Die*, I experimented with eliminating meat and dairy from my diet. Three months later, my cholesterol dropped to normal levels and I no longer needed medications. After going on a plant-based diet, all my [many other] issues disappeared [too] and I felt more vibrant than ever. That was when I realized the power of our choices.

Like Juan, I believe everything is interrelated. Eating habits that are not in sync with nature and the planet cannot properly support our health.

The bottom line is, we need to treat our bodies as our temples and to recognize that for every action, there is a reaction. That goes for pretty much anything you consume. Make sure you pick those foods that will lead to the most positive outcomes for your mind, your body and your spirit.

‖‖

Give It a Try:
Find Your Sweet Spot in a Minute

Our society thrives on quick fixes. For some, that means caffeine, burgers, booze, smoking or recreational or unnecessary drugs. The longer the habit, the harder it is to release.

Chaitanya has a three-tiered approach to break free from those crutches.

1. Awareness:
   Be aware of the consequences of all your actions, positive and negative. Those magic moments when you are consuming unhealthy substances, even if they seem harmless, like drinking a few glasses of wine with dinner, can have negative repercussions. Some adverse health consequences can arise quickly in abusing certain substances, while others creep up and catch you by surprise.

2. Alternatives:
   Welcome alternatives rather than getting stuck in a rut with unhealthy routines. We are creatures of habit. It is hard to give up one without developing another. Find something good to replace the bad.

   Imagine a Venn diagram with overlapping circles. Fill one with the behavior you want to modify. In the second, add what is good for you. The intersection of the two circles is the sweet spot. Find what you like *and* what is good for you. For example, if you like wine and know fruit is healthier, the sweet spot can be fruit juice with sparkling water.

3. Association:
Associate with those who support healthy choices. If you're trying to stop smoking, stay far from smokers. If you're trying to stop drinking, find alcohol-free social scenes.

While that doesn't mean you have to cut off family and friends, connecting with people with positive lifestyles reinforces your resolution to maintain a healthy one yourself.

It's common for parents to scrutinize who their children socialize with. Oftentimes, we encourage our school-age kids to participate in sports, music or other activities to keep them away from potentially harmful environments.

We are social creatures who want to fit in. As responsible adults, it requires great inner strength to say "no" when you are surrounded by smokers or drinkers. Take the shortcut. Avoid those situations where you know there will be overindulging.

In summary, a pure and harmonious sattvic lifestyle nourishes our mind, body and spirit. Now let's explore another age-old tradition that brings us balance: the day of rest.

Chapter 8: Shabbat as Your Reboot in the Digital Age

Shabbat is truly a gift to humanity.

—Rabbi Sarah Schechter

Most of us move on autopilot and often lack clarity in our thoughts and intentions. The lightning-paced speed at which we try to get things done only causes chaos and roadblocks. Taking periodic breaks recharges the mind, body and spirit. The ancient practice of *Shabbat*,[115] or the day of rest, is the reboot we need.

My grandparents were Eastern European Jews who escaped from the pogroms and forced ghetto life before WWII began. My ethnicity is Jewish, but I have scant experience with the religion. We were secular Jews, and yet my mother beamed with pride when my cousin Joe married Rabbi Sarah Schechter.

Though Sarah is neither my rabbi nor a blood relative, she is a kindred spirit with much knowledge to share. Sarah has a knack for making things easy to understand. She passes on her wisdom in a kaffeeklatsch manner. No preaching. No shaming. Just simple expressions of "here's what it's all about."

A doctoral candidate, Chaplain Major Schechter is the first female rabbi to serve in the United States Air Force (USAF). At one point, Rabbi Sarah served near me at Lackland Air Force Base in San Antonio, Texas. She invited me to a beautiful *Sukkot* (festival for the harvest) ceremony that she coordinated and led. People of all races and religions, including an Islamic imam and a Catholic priest, sat elbow to elbow on white folding chairs at tables covered in paper tablecloths inside a three-sided *sukkah* (open-air autumnal hut). Designed and installed by Rabbi Sarah, the white tent, adorned with pine and palm, represented the temporary booths in which our ancestors lived in the wilderness.

The handcrafted sukkah seemed out of place in the middle of that huge airbase. Inside the structure, we were all one, celebrating the customs and traditions passed down from the Holy Land. Whether Jew or gentile, servicemen or civilian, religious or secular, young or old, all shared the opportunity to learn from my cousin, the rabbi.

This chapter features advice from Rabbi Sarah that's appropriate for everyone, from when she served as Branch Chief of Plans and Programs at Ramstein Air Base in Germany. Unlike what you might expect, Rabbi Sarah's guidance is accessible to all, regardless of one's belief in God.

The Rabbi in Combat Boots: Sarah Schechter

Raised in Greenwich Village, Sarah was a vocal student at the Fiorello H. Laguardia High School of Music and Performing Arts. Laguardia is better known as "the Fame school," featured in the 1980s musical. It has a long list of celebrity alumni, including actors Al Pacino and Jennifer Aniston, singer Nicki Minaj, and *Saturday Night Live's* Michael Che.

Changes of scenery, scripts, sets and wardrobes are part of Sarah's life. The active-duty chaplain is comfortable in Air Force fatigues, combat boots, a flak jacket, or with a *yarmulke* (Jewish head covering), prayer shawl, long-sleeved top, and ankle-length skirt.

Sarah swapped the performance arena to immerse herself in foreign languages in college. She earned an undergrad degree in Hebrew and Jewish Studies from Hunter College and a second degree in Japanese.

She was intrigued by Jewish history in Japan. As part of her undergraduate work, she spent a year on a kibbutz in Israel and even more time in Kyoto and Kobe investigating the Jewish community in Japan. With her proficiency and passion for the Japanese language, the Japanese telephone company NTT hired her as an interpreter after graduation.

At home in New York, Israel or Japan, Sarah felt something was missing from her career, but she could not put her finger on it. Her mother, an award-winning gemstone carver and goldsmith who often thought outside of the box, had the answer. Sarah's mom suggested her personality would be fitting to follow in her father's footsteps and attend rabbinical school.

Sarah felt the advice was worth investigating and chose to attend the Hebrew Union College-Jewish Institute of Religion, the oldest rabbinical seminary in the United States. She met her soon-to-be husband, Joe, while living and studying in Los Angeles.

Two years before her ordination, tragedy struck. The attacks on the World Trade Center and the Pentagon shocked the native New Yorker. Sarah's career path became crystal clear. She had an immediate desire to support servicepeople, who dedicate their lives to protect our nation, and their families, who make so many sacrifices of their own.

In an interview with the Air Force News Service,[116] Sarah said:

> Within seconds of the attack on our country, the military suddenly stopped being an undefined culture I was vaguely familiar with and their mission became absolutely clear—protection of our country, protection of our loved ones, and protection of our very lives. I felt a great sense of compassion toward our service members. I knew they carried a huge burden on their shoulders, and I wanted, as a Jew and as a future rabbi, to stand shoulder to shoulder with them.

The day after the 9/11 attacks, the rabbinical student called the United States Air Force to offer her pastoral services to the military community.

In a USAF recruiting video,[117] she stated:

> That morning, all I wanted to do was to let our service members know there were many of us out there who support them and wanted to help them feel confident in the job they were doing. I would gladly give back my experiences here [with the USAF] for September 11th to have never happened. But I am grateful I'm able to have this experience, and it's opened my eyes up to a whole other culture.

As a USAF chaplain, Rabbi Schechter responds to the call of duty anywhere in the world. Trained in protection against chemical weaponry and other specialized tactics, the rabbi serves the military community of all faiths, even in the most dangerous combat locations. In a farewell letter to her deployed unit, the rabbi wrote these words from the Book of Ruth.

Wherever you go, I will go; where you lodge, I will lodge; your people shall be my people, and your God my God. And where you die, I will die.

Stateside, she has crisscrossed the country fulfilling multiyear assignments. Among them, she served as chaplain to the Presidential Airlift Group of Air Force One and Two at Andrews Air Base in Maryland, the United States Air Force Academy in Colorado, and the USAF Reserve Command Headquarters in Georgia.

"Major," "rabbi," "chaplain" and "doctor" are just titles. Although she is usually wearing her camouflage uniform, Sarah is more than just one of the troops. She is a spiritual leader, counselor, teacher, community-builder and confidant—in addition to being a wife and mother.

Rabbi Sarah reads Hebrew verses from the *bimah* (pulpit) while adding ample explanations in English to invite people of all faiths to share in the teachings, rituals, traditions and celebrations. She builds bridges between diverse representatives in our military community. Likewise, she serves as a link between the spiritual world and the day-to-day pressures of combat life, separated families, physical wounds, and other triggers that wear away at the enlisted and their loved ones.

As she told the Air Force News Service:

Strong relationships and active participation in a caring community are absolutely vital to spiritual as well as physical wellness.

The Guru's Wisdom: Turn Shabbat into a Weekly Retreat

Even as a young child, Sarah knew that a day of rest was beautiful and special. Recognizing one day a week as different from the other six days was part of her family's lifestyle. The practice of holy rest for the spirit to be refreshed is something she deems vital.

> Shabbat is a gift to those who keep it, Jewish or not Jewish, through community, through prayer, through singing, through eating, through loving, through rest—and repeating.

Wherever this US Air Force chaplain is in the world, Friday night is special. She shares the gift of Shabbat. The Sabbath is a time for human and holy connections.

Believing that the twenty-five-hour period from sundown Friday until after sundown Saturday is a sacred time to be inclusive, inviting and hospitable, she creates a home away from home for all.

In Rabbi Sarah's words:

> The beauty of the community Joe and I have built is that many of the wonderful souls who regularly join us for Shabbat happen to be deeply devoted followers of their own faith traditions—Christianity, Islam, Sikhism and Vaishnavism. Occasionally, a neo-pagan or a Native American stops by. Even people of no faith orientation, who simply live by the ideals and idealism of humanism, share in our sacred time, song, study and meal. Our Friday evening Sabbath serves as a place and a platform to welcome people of all faiths, all races, all politi-

cal viewpoints, and all sexual orientations so they may learn from and grow with each other.

To paint a clearer picture of the 3,000-year-old tradition, the rabbi explains the literal meaning of *Shabbat*, which is to "stop," "cease" or "rest." The Torah tells us, "Shabbat vayinafash," which essentially means stop, rest and be refreshed. *Nafash* is related to the word *nefesh* (soul). In other words, says Rabbi Sarah, "Stop. Be refreshed. Nourish your soul. This is the gift of Shabbat, and the brilliance of Judaism."

Before the invention of the light bulb, active life was primarily sunrise to sunset. When our ancestors worked six long days every week, it was a different era. There were no devices to connect people with their coworkers, clients or bosses 24/7. No one had any inclination to travel hundreds or thousands of miles at high speed for a business meeting or a weekend getaway.

The increased intensity of modern working lifestyles in the last generation swung to more days and longer hours—all the more reason to hold a sacred time to stop, be refreshed, and focus on the soul.

> You have to unplug from the material to plug into that which is infinite. Today's world is run, run, run. [There are so] many distractions. The bigger question is, what are we running from? What is today's distraction that I need to run to, so I can run [away] from where I genuinely need to be? From antiquity, within Judaism, Shabbat was a radical realization that there are times we simply need to devote ourselves to *being*—being in prayer, being in family, being in community, and being centered.

Rabbi Schechter invites people to welcome the treasures of the Sabbath and focus on all that is positive, to praise God or a higher being for everything in your life. This follows in line with the Sabbath liturgy, which admonishes us to refrain from complaining.

Shabbat is said to give those who observe it a glimpse of the Messianic era. According to Rabbi Schechter:

> No more hunger, loneliness or war. Shabbat is a taste of peace and harmony in the most profound sense imaginable, *if* we surrender into her (Shabbat).

The sacred day of stopping helps us to carve out time for introspection or the Almighty.

Rabbi Schechter likens keeping the Sabbath to what she calls "kosher living." Just as kosher dietary laws involve healthy restrictions on diet, the same is true for Shabbat in defining healthy limitations concerning work. With no restrictions, the norm could be more chaotic for individuals, society and the environment. Kosher living is a mindset that contributes to physical, mental and spiritual balance and well-being.

Rabbi Schechter notes that restraining ourselves just one day out of seven:

> ...uniquely opens up other avenues and opportunities for us to hear the inner call of our soul. The root of our being cries out: seek, encounter and surrender to that which nourishes all of existence.

The practice of honoring the Sabbath encourages disconnecting from anything that is distracting or not conducive to a Shabbat environment. Traditional Jewish religious law prohibits thirty-nine major categories of activities on the day of rest, including driving, riding and using modern conveniences. However, a more secular approach encourages you to just turn off electronic devices. Appreciate and protect that sacred day in the manner that is right for you—with no complaints and no judgment.

Rabbi Sarah's Five Easy Tips

1. **Take baby steps in changing your lifestyle.**
   A beautiful way to begin is by incorporating a special Friday night dinner into your schedule. Then, choose to turn off your phone and computer, one day each week. For example, carve out special time for uninterrupted meditation or communing with nature.

2. **Light up your life.**
   Light candles to signal the start of your Sabbath practice. The radiant light of the flickering flames throughout the house is a peaceful, beautiful and traditional reminder that you can spark sacred peace and love in your life and your family's.

3. **Remember that this day is different.**
   Beyond lighting candles as a marker of the beginning of the observance, find ways to inspire sacredness in the next twenty-five hours. The Sabbath is not for business-as-usual. Engage in sacred thought, speech and deed that root, reinforce and realize the spirit of Shabbat.

4. **Recognize blessing and refrain from complaining.**
   Whether you choose a traditional twenty-five-hour Shabbat, a digital detox, or a secular Sabbath, seek to see the beauty and grace in all things. Over time, this

practice may influence how you walk through life the other six days of the week.

5. **Connect to a higher being.**
Regardless of your faith background or affiliation, use this day of rest to reflect on what is enduring, both beyond and within. Connect to the Supreme or simply to existence itself. Remember, we are minor players in this galaxy of infinite wisdom.

Shabbat as a Weekly Reboot

Back when I was entrenched in the corporate world, I worked seven days a week, around the clock. During one job interview, my future boss made it clear Type-A team players filled the cubicles. He quipped that working half-days meant logging twelve hours each day.

For many years, it was not uncommon for me to get out of bed at 3 a.m., power up my computer, and respond to emails, strategize marketing plans, or draft editorial content.

At another workplace, one of my colleagues stressed the importance of being on call. She even carried her cell phone into the bathroom—just in case. Mind you, we were not emergency room nurses, first responders or firefighters. My cohorts and I promoted sales of big-name products and services. It was nothing that couldn't wait a few minutes, hours or even days.

I was what my company called "a road-warrior." Before virtual meetings became part of standard operating procedures, I often spent upward of eight hours in transit for a one-hour meeting, with no time for sightseeing or even a decent meal.

The norm was to hop on the 6 or 7 a.m. flight out, connect to another plane who-knows-where, and eat a snack in the rental car headed to an early afternoon meeting. If I was lucky, presentations and discussions would end in time to catch an early evening return flight. That meant buying airport popcorn or a bag of nuts as dinner and getting home around midnight. Then I was back in the home office early the next morning.

Those long hours in-flight were not spent reading a novel, watching a movie, or meditating. More often than not, I was preparing conference reports, editing content, and updating timelines.

On vacations, when I did not bring my laptop, I headed to communal computer rental rooms in India, Ecuador, Turkey, Poland or wherever to keep in touch. The big challenge was locating the @ sign on foreign keyboards.

After I left the corporate world, I recognized the benefits of slowing down. I unplugged long before bedtime to improve sleep patterns. All my televisions, stereos and VHS, CD and DVD players went to Goodwill. I cut my dependence on my MacBook Pro, but my iPhone was my everything. It was my messenger, alarm clock, timer, music player, guided meditation source, camera, calculator, flashlight, newspaper and connection to friends and family. I began stashing the smartphone in another room a few hours before going to bed. I muted my ringer and activated the "do not disturb" to avoid hearing the pinging of alerts. That helped. But it was not enough.

Joanna, my high-strung sister, calls me "Miss Namaste." Yet, my longtime Ayurvedic doctor detected I had more work to do. Underneath my calm persona were frazzled nerves. I needed to shut down more often to recharge.

My doctor gave me his interpretation of the Genesis passage, "On the seventh day, [God] rested."[118] He quipped, "God didn't rest. The universe would fall apart if she did. But we should."

That was my wake-up call. I incorporated Shabbat into my Ayurvedic regime. One day a week, I refrain from driving (or riding) in any vehicle, plane or train, and all my electronic or digital devices are silenced and out of reach. I distance myself from the hubbub and surround myself with yoga, meditation, nature and other forms of self-care and reflection.

At first, I could not imagine getting through a full twenty-four hours without my cell phone. Now, I cherish my special day.

My Ayurvedic doctor suggested extended disconnects of three to seven days a few times a year. In fact, the concept of this book arose during my first seventy-two-hour, solo, Sabbath silent retreat.

The Power of Unplugging

Anne Lamott is a well-known San Francisco Bay Area author, Guggenheim Fellowship recipient, and longtime Sunday school teacher. In one of her books, with her trademark frankness and wry humor, she says the solution to most problems is to just unplug for a few minutes, including ourselves.

Tiffany Shlain is another Northern California-based bestselling author who confirms the value of a day of rest in her book *24/6: The Power of Unplugging One Day a Week*. An Emmy-nominated filmmaker and founder of the Webby Awards, she says slowing down takes you farther. Shlain, her husband, their two daughters, her employees, and countless friends acknowledge they need to unplug periodically to gear back up with more power and creativity. Shlain calls this a "Tech Shabbat."

In *24/6*, she shares many tips about how to join the Sabbath-holders' bandwagon in the seemingly impossible-to-disconnect world in which we live. She affirms the practice is ideal for enhanced productivity, but also social interaction and familial relationships.

Irene Michaels explored the holistic health benefits of unplugging in the context of Shabbat for her master's thesis at St. Catherine University.[119]

A registered nurse and holistic health coach, Michaels says:

> Some would say that we have lost our human connection to each other and ourselves, despite being electronically connected to everything and anything. In reviewing the literature on the health effects from overuse of technology, I came to believe that we need to find a way to take a break from this pseudoconnection and return to human interactions without an electronic intermediary.

Michaels points to research that confirms the negative effects of over-stimulation and information overload. Our reliance and addictions to electronic and digital media damage our physical and mental health. As a result of the social media craze, our interpersonal relationships suffer.

Between 1985 and 2004, the number of Americans who considered themselves socially isolated tripled.[120] The COVID-19 pandemic spiked feelings of intense loneliness. But those emotions weren't fleeting. According to studies in 2021, 79 percent of American adults aged eighteen to twenty-four feel lonely and 42 percent in the eighteen to thirty-four age group reported "always" feeling "left out."[121]

According to an article by the American Academy of Ophthalmology, 61 percent of Americans admit to being addicted to the internet and their devices. Those spending more time online are 2.5 times more likely to experience depression.[122]

Michaels evaluated six observant Jewish women who limited electronic devices one day a week. The researcher's unique style of data collection was through words and photographs that the participants recorded in journals and collages. The output from the health coach's technique, called "Soulcollage," yielded positive commonalities.

> From the interviews and discussions of images, seven themes emerged: mental relief, social connection, self-care, [appreciation of] nature, spiritual community, stress [relief], and [respect for] spirituality. The majority of statements by the participants expressed a feeling of peace and serenity... Being unplugged regularly on Shabbat was like a spa for your brain... Participants repeatedly used common words, such as "peaceful," "calm," "relaxation," "stillness" and "relief." All the participants made statements emphasizing the importance of being in nature. Without the connection to their cell phones, they spoke of feeling tuned into the rhythm of nature.

Barbara Baker Speedling, also a St. Catherine University grad student, tracked ten women raised as Christians in her thesis "Celebrating Sabbath: An Organic Inquiry into the Transformative Power of a Sanctuary in Time."[123]

The Celebrating Sabbath respondents represented a broad cultural cross section: five Caucasians, one African American, one Hispanic, one Italian American, a Filipina American, and one Swede. The women did not all adhere to the orthodox practice of Shabbat, but crafted what worked best for them, their households, and within their community. Participants agreed the day of rest allowed them to be more present in their relationships and more considerate of others.

Baker Speedling's research found six common themes.

> Sabbath-keeping enhances self-awareness, improves self-care, enriches relationships, develops spirituality, and positively impacts the rest of a participant's week.

The sixth commonality between the female research participants was that they each acknowledged that their Sabbath-keeping practices and philosophies evolved over time.

While Baker Speedling never asked participants about their opinions observing the Sabbath on a larger scale, they each suggested society would be better off if a day of rest was the norm.

Similar to what Shlain notes in her book 24/6, one respondent said the Sabbath day helps her "go from overwhelmed to energized." She feels a change in power dynamics and closer to God. Another said Sabbath was a day to "reground, repurpose and reflect."

Baker Speedling summarizes her results.

> Sabbath is a sacred gift from our Jewish sisters and brothers. Reviving the best parts of this ancient tradition can be an antidote to many modern-day stresses. Sabbath-keeping is a powerful, cost-effective, holistic practice that can contribute significantly to all aspects of our well-being... It is accessible to almost anyone and requires no special tools or training.

Plus, Sabbath-keeping contributes to our ecosystem. When you disconnect, you reconnect with nature, creating respect for the environment, and by refraining from driving or riding in vehicles, trains, buses or planes, we help offset the carbon footprint.

The benefits of a digital disconnect far outweigh missing your social media feeds or an unending string of emails. All it takes is prioritizing your sense of what is important. Disconnect from the artificial and connect to the natural by adding Shabbat to your routine.

||||||||||||||||||||||||||||||||||||||||||||||||||||||||||||||||||||||||||||||||||||||||||||||||||||||||||||||||||||||||||||||||||||||||

Give It a Try:
Disconnect Your Devices

1. Choose your start date.

   As with any change in habit, the hardest part is to make the decision. Set a date to begin and stick with it.

2. Design your detox.

   Choose what is doable. Determine which hours or days you will practice your disconnect and what you will limit and replace. Choose options that best fit your social and work life. Just like diets allow you to swap out foods, give yourself leeway to change when needed.

3. Give people a heads up.

   Let others know about your disconnect so they are aware of why you are not picking up the phone or responding to texts or emails. Ask housemates, spouses or live-in partners to be supportive. Better yet, invite them to join in with the digital detox.

4. Use technology to your advantage.

   Set your smartphones to "do not disturb" and program "screen time" limitations. Find more tips and inspiration at awayfortheday.org or digitaldetox.com.

5. Enjoy the sacred day.

Replace the hours you spend on your devices with quality time among friends and family, luxuriate in self-care, or relish the silence.

Getting close to nature is a powerful spiritual booster too. My next guru shares ways to honor and connect with God's garden.

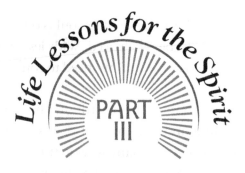

PART
III

Beyond the Visible

Young children can point to the head and different body parts, but drawing a picture of the soul is an abstract work of art. I think of expressionist Marc Chagall's angel-like figures that seem to float among clouds. He is heavy on the smoky grays and blues that give his paintings an ethereal feel.

When I was a kid, I took piano lessons. My teacher had health issues, so she was a no-show more often than not. I never became a virtuoso, but I could play Hoagy Carmichael's "Heart and Soul." It was a very simple song with just a few notes played in almost an arrhythmic manner. Bing. Bing. Bing. Badum, badum, badum. At least, that's how I played it.

To this day, when I think of the soul, I think of the emotions or intelligence that emanate from the heart. Our society trains us to be led by our brains. We discount our instincts and true nature so much that the heart and spirit take back seats.

Picture the brain as the conductor. The body is the precious instrument like a Stradivarius or a Steinway grand piano. The soul is the musician who creates the work of art. Each element is essential. Working in harmony creates magic.

Pianos and violins need tune-ups, and maestros refine their craft to produce a masterpiece. Our brains, bodies and spirits need attention too. Since the spirit or soul is often overlooked, the equation needs to be rebalanced. With less attention and understanding given to the soul, we need to connect it to loud-speakers.

The spirit is our connection to nature, to the Creator, to love and understanding, and to humankind. It is our essence and our true being. There are so many ways to tune in and tune up the spirit. Some may resonate with you today. Others may feel perfect next year. Go with your gut feeling, which is usually your soul talking.

Chapter 9: Connection with the Creator and the Universe

Mother Earth is my church.

—Gloria Camarillo Vasquez

Gloria Camarillo Vasquez is a Texas native who treasures her tribal heritage. She is an elder with the Tap Pilam Coahuiltecan Nation, a tribal community whose clans spread from South Texas to San Luis Potosí, Mexico. In 1990, she and her family formed a nonprofit called "American Indians in Texas at the Spanish Colonial Missions," which strives to restore the dignity and well-being of the people and the land through love, respect and trust for Indigenous values.

A live television broadcast of *Good Morning America* introduced me to Gloria. The show was a big deal for my client, the San Antonio Convention and Visitor's Bureau. With a flick of a switch, one hundred twenty-two thousand lights sparkled along the River Walk to signal the start of the holiday season. Over the span of two hours, a montage of engaging interviews highlighted our city's cultural heritage. Televised scenes vanish in the blink of an eye, but the *Good Morning America* segments required months of preparation and hundreds of crew members.

I was one of the first people on the set. It was about 4:30 a.m. when I met the effervescent Gloria; her granddaughter snuggled on her lap. Not ready for the bright lights, microphones and cameras of her national television debut, nine-year-old Bella's live shot was from a pop-up kitchen squeezed between a string of dozens of colorful umbrellas atop round, outdoor café tables. By 6:00 a.m., the young girl was all smiles, hand-patting cornmeal *masa*[124] into shape to demonstrate tamale-making to the world.

About a month later, Gloria and I worked behind the scenes for a live broadcast of another television network. More recently, we joined forces for the first-ever National Basketball Association Indigenous Night. The San Antonio Spurs paid homage to Native cultures across the globe and introduced the Tap Pilam Coahuiltecan Nation to millions via several live television segments.

Native spirituality and healing are the sources of Gloria's inner strength and resilient nature. Anyone can practice her lessons about connecting to the Creator of all living things.

The Native Elder: Gloria Camarillo Vasquez

Things were not always easy for Gloria. At just thirteen, she took on adult responsibilities by looking after her seven siblings. Later, at the height of her professional career, she faced racial discrimination in the workplace. Never one to stay quiet, she filed a lawsuit even though her employer was a major branch of the federal government that evokes fear in most people. But fear was not on Gloria's agenda.

> All my life, I honored prayer and faith, yet kept a
> machete in my hand. The lawsuit was a big fight

> against a lot of people with a lot of power—corporate and governmental. But I had willpower and faith and my ancestral resistance. I was not going to give up. They were discriminating, not only against me, but others.

This confident woman was willing to do whatever needed to be done to take a stand. When she first complained about the prejudices to her boss, the response was "Get used to it." Gloria knew there was no chance of accepting the discrimination, so she filed eighteen complaints and fifteen union grievances. A judge in Washington, DC, ruled in her favor.

When she thinks back, she considers those two life tests as minor-league hurdles compared to when she left her husband of ten years. Gloria headed 1,300 miles north to stay with a sister in Milwaukee. She did not catch a nonstop flight with complimentary drinks and snacks. Nor was she in an SUV with video players. She hopped on a Greyhound with three suitcases and three kids under the age of seven. Her belongings shared space in the youngest child's case.

She recalls those days like it was yesterday.

> I signed my divorce papers on a Wednesday. On Thursday, I got on the bus. It was something I had to do. It was the only way I knew how to get ahead in life. I was taught resilience; to be the best I could be. My maternal grandpa was an entrepreneur. My father's father worked in the fields from sunup to sundown.

Her spiritual guides, faith, prayer and ancestral practices subdued any fear and intimidation.

> I am a privileged woman because I stand on the shoulders of powerful women. My grandmothers

were *guerreras* (fighters), resistors whose blood runs through my veins. They taught me to face and conquer obstacles and appreciate my blessings.

It was the time of the civil rights movement. Gloria landed a job within a month of her move as director of an inner-city development project. The quick-thinking, outspoken high school graduate became responsible for an anti-poverty program serving Milwaukee's Mexican community. The challenge she faced when she was just thirteen and helping her family was now a blessing.

> Leaving Texas with nothing, I saw a large salary of $10,000 a year and excitedly said, "I'll take it." Little did I know that having to take care of my brothers and sisters would prepare me for being the boss of people with college degrees, because it taught me how to lead.

The single mom led the social service agency for three years, all while recognizing her potential for an even brighter future if she had a college degree.

> I was raised to earn life's rewards. I have never felt inferior to anybody or anything. No. I'm going to get to where I'm going because of my abilities, strengths and endurance.

The self-reliant woman was not interested in handouts or shortcuts. She did not apply for any scholarships or social service benefits. Life's successes were going to be based on her own merits. She paid the full tuition and juggled school, work and home responsibilities.

She enrolled in social work courses at Milwaukee Area Technical School, where she scored all A's. Just one year there gave her the push she needed to apply to the prestigious Jesuit-run private school, Marquette University.

When she confided her goal of trading up to a private four-year college to a colleague, he was not impressed, saying, "Jefa (boss lady), you can't teach old dogs new tricks."

She laughed off his comment and lit her candles, offered prayers to her Creator and burned sage, believing "Neglecting spiritual well-being weakens the state of mind."

Gloria's dream school said "yes." She was thirty-nine, more than twice the age of the other co-eds.

> The first day of school, I sat under a tree and cried, but I told myself I had to keep going. The only brown face I could see was me and a couple of African American children. I got up from sitting under the tree, cleaned my skirt, and said to myself, "Let's go." I never missed classes. In the snow. In the rain. It was a beautiful experience in my life.

A few years later, her résumé listed a dual degree, with one major in sociology and another in criminology and law. Gloria gives credit to her Creator for a strong spirit, which was her anchor to survive life's rocky roads.

"How the Creator helped me! I was always with my little altar and prayer," she says, referring to her home shrine decorated with images of her ancestors, crucifixes and other sacred symbols.

Today, Gloria enjoys leading opening prayers at civic events and teaching students of all ages. She served as an in-house resident healer at Stanford University and was the source of curricula content at Evergreen Valley College in San Jose, California. At the San Antonio Missions, she is an ambassador to young students visiting from the United States and Canada who are interested in Native American traditions.

The Guru's Wisdom: Honor Your Ancestors

Gloria was raised with Indigenous, spiritism and Catholic beliefs. Her spiritual practices are a special blend that dates back many generations.

> My *Guachichil*[125] ancestors didn't idolize gods but revered the sun and the moon. Honoring Mother Moon is a family tradition taught by *apa* (dad) who learned from his apa. My apa was a man of *palabra* (his word) and of so many talents. Apa not only told us stories about beautiful and intriguing Mother Moon and the stars, but he also taught us how to pray. To this day, I pray in Spanish and receive Mother Moon messages. The warm and beautiful evenings in *las colonias del* (the neighborhoods of) West Side in San Antonio felt like paradise. Mother Moon adorned the universe with radiant rays of light, millions of shining stars, and the sky so blue.

Some seventy years later, her father's presence is still strong. Her daily routine includes morning spiritual prayers of gratitude for seeing another sunrise. A visionary person, she heeds the messages from the spiritual guides of her ancestors and passes on the teachings to the next generations within and outside of her bloodlines. Most important, her ancestral practices are universal and can be adopted by anyone regardless of their age, socioeconomic level, geography or heritage.

Following are her three key revelations.

First, the universe is the source of our spiritual, emotional and physical well-being. We just need to know how to tap into its abundance and generosity.

> We all have the ability to connect to God, the Creator, the universe. Together, and among all living things, we are the universe. We have the power because we are his creation, and he is within us and we are within him. Set up an altar or special sacred space to praise and give thanks to our Creator for all the revelations and lessons given to us.

Second, open up to the spirit world.

> I was taught to bless myself as soon as I woke up— to go to the altar, give thanks to God, our Creator, and ask my spiritual ancestral protectors for a productive day and to protect me from all harm.

> Our ancestors guide us here on earth. They are our spiritual protectors and our teachers. Faith takes us along our path. The spirits of our ancestors lead us to come up with answers to address the steps we need to take to overcome obstacles.

Her third lesson teaches us that true wealth comes from one's connection to the Creator or spirituality. People should love and protect their thoughts, their bodies and, above all, their spirit.

Gloria explains:

> Spiritual enfoldment leads to the epitome of happiness. Whether one is rich or poor, it is possible to obtain that happiness because it's a spiritual fulfillment that is not connected to material things.

Birth is a blessing and a gift to enjoy our earthly journey, keeping in mind that we are here for spiritual perfection. We learn to have reverence for Mother Earth and be grateful for all she provides for our growth and basic needs, like water, food and shelter.

Spiritual enfoldment evolves through good deeds and actions toward others and connecting with our Creator's creations.

Gloria's time-honored teachings value humbleness, balanced with courage and strength. Love and respect for life were handed down from her elders as easy and beautiful customs to incorporate into her lifestyle. No guidebook is needed. No magic potions. No anointed leader, helpers or inaccessible house of prayer. The location is wherever you are. The ingredients are the most basic found in nature. The words are those that resonate with your heart.

I visit my altar as soon as I get up. I wash my hands and bless myself and the rocks on my altar with my sacred moon water. I give thanks to my Creator. I ask permission to invoke the spirits of my grandmothers, and I ask for my children and myself to be surrounded by white light for protection.

She notes her prayers come from within in contrast to scripted Catholic litanies like "Hail Mary." Her supplications are spontaneous words of love and compassion.

I don't need a building, nor anyone's permission to pray. Prayer is within me. The words that come out of me, they're not written anywhere. It might be four words or four sentences. For example, I might pray, "Creator, may I always remember to give more than I take." What I say depends on the moment and my connection with the Creator. When it comes from my spirit, I am a mass of energy filled with reverence and gratitude.

Her respect for life continues beyond her sunrise routine. Three times a day, she goes outside and prays to the earth and the universe. Her sanctuary is her garden. Mother Nature is her church.

Gloria's grandmothers passed on their knowledge of natural healing remedies and traditions to her, which she deems necessary and useful answers for life's survival. Now, she brings these cultural gifts to another three generations of her descendants.

She extracts some of her curative blends right from her garden. She grows rue, a strong medicinal herb. While basil is a fine seasoning, Gloria uses the herb for light *limpias* (a spiritual cleansing). She cuts from her aloe vera plant to soothe burns and itches with its salve. One of Gloria's favorite recipes is to take the spinnings from spider webs and carefully rub them on small cuts. This is nature's Band-Aid with no ouch factor when you pull it off. The silky sticky white threads are soft enough for babies.

Gloria doesn't need artificial stimulants or unhealthy depressants in her medicine cabinet. She taps into natural, cost-free sources with no contraindications to rev up or wind down. Here are a few examples.

I boost my energy by meditating with beautiful rocks I collected from the area where my Guachi-chil ancestors lived in Zacatecas, Mexico.

> As I caress the rocks, I pray and envision my ances-
> tors, their beautiful bodies decorated with red
> paint—their favorite color—and their warrior
> *danza* (dance) boosting their energy levels by their
> feet touching these same blessed rocks I hold in
> my hands.
>
> When I open my eyes, my heart rate is soaring. My
> hands are pulsating, and my whole body is vibrat-
> ing with electrifying energy. The blood and energy
> of my ancestors flow through my body and con-
> tinue to flow through my children's children.

Just as a baby falls asleep rocking in a cradle, Gloria uses the
soothing qualities of water instead of sleeping pills. She picked
up this practice from her parents and grandmother when she
lived near an Air Force base. During her childhood, sirens
blasted at all hours, aircraft hovered overhead, and bomb
drills were the norm. Pleasant dreams were not automatic.

The trick to peaceful slumber became a ritual. She places a
glass of water, which is one of the elements that attracts negative energy, under her bed below her head. In the morning, she
pours the water outside to the east, where the new day begins.

She explains:

> We are made of water, which finds a way as energy
> to rock us to sleep. It soothes us. It sways us back
> and forth. Water is like a sponge. It soaks up neg-
> ativity.

Full moons are opportunities for special prayers. Gloria's spontaneous lunar recitations may sound something like this:

> Queen of the night, lighting my path, I pray
> for peace and protection for all of us. May your

magical manifestation touch every one of us to be the best we can be as we walk along our earthly path.

Gloria Vasquez's Five Easy Tips

1. Find your sacred space.
   Set up an altar or small space in your home, ideally facing east to represent new beginnings. The area does not have to be elaborate or large. Even a tiny corner in your home is sufficient. Decorate the dedicated spot with photos of ancestors, teachers, spiritual guides, gods or goddesses, or holy symbols, like a rosary.

2. Absorb the light within.
   Light a candle and place it on your altar as you say a prayer. There is no right or wrong way, as long as the intention is pure. Gloria anoints a small votive candle with olive oil as she gives thanks to the Creator. She visualizes positive thoughts related to what she wants to manifest. She "dresses" the candle by poking around the wick with a tiny stick to represent the cardinal directions and rubs frankincense, cedar oil or healing herbs around the top. After the candle is prepared, she places it in her sacred space, lights the flame, and lets the votive burn out on its own.

3. Tap into Mother Moon's powerful energy with moon water.
   Prepare your moon water every night. (Instructions are in the "Give It a Try" section on page 171.) Use the water to anoint yourself. Bless your house by sprinkling the moon water throughout your living space. Add a drop or two to your teacup or pour some in your bathwater.

4. Fill your home with life.

Place plants outside your front door and throughout your home, including your bedroom. It is optimal to have greenery that faces the east to greet the new day. Consider growing aloe vera, which cuts through negative energy and attracts abundance.

5. Give more than you take.

Respect people, traditions and the planet. Nurture others. Share your knowledge. Pray for others. Plant seeds, literally and figuratively. We are just a speck in the universe.

Returning to Native Ancestral Traditions

One of my rituals is connecting to the spiritual world before I write. I light a scented candle and palo santo[126] or sage. I place them near an 8″ x 10″ black-and-white studio graduation portrait of my mother. Her name was Gloria. Before my fingers start to type, I gaze into her eyes and ask to receive her creativity and literary expertise. She was a writer and my first (and most important) writing coach.

That special image of my mom is not at my altar. It is just a make-shift sacred space at my work desk. My altar is in my meditation room. There, I have smaller sepia-toned framed pictures of my parents and grandparents. One rock sits alongside the images. The rock came from my aunt's garden. At her memorial, I hand-painted it in uplifting colors with the date she had passed away.

I adopted the sacred spaces and practices after my mother died and Gloria Vasquez entered my life. However, I have always been drawn to and valued the traditions and spirituality of Indigenous people. I chose to live and work in countries rich with Indigenous customs and languages.

The following are two instances where I witnessed the healing power of ancestral traditions.

I lived high in the Andes when I was pregnant with my daughter and for the first two years of her life. At around eighteen months, she ate little. We took her to the head of the children's hospital. His diagnosis was *susto*, a temporary emotional or spiritual scare or traumatic experience. His prescription: *una limpia*. I trusted him and wanted him to heal her. He declined, saying he was a doctor. We needed to find a *curandera*.[127]

We found a practicing healer in one of the stalls of the bustling central market who offered her services in the aisle between towering stacks of herbs. As she rubbed my daughter all over with the magic cure, she muttered healing phrases in Quechua, the language of the Indigenous peoples of the Andes. She also gave us home remedies to continue for a few weeks. We added flowers to our baby's bathwater and fed her something that looked like long blades of grass. I knew a dose of chlorophyll is healthy, so I wasn't concerned. My rational mind accepted the science behind the spiritual traditions.

My tiny daughter thrived.

Thirty years later, I continue practices similar to those prescribed by the marketplace curandera. My Ayurvedic doctor wants me to soak in hot water infused with essential oils for thirty minutes every night—not unlike the flowers in my baby's tub. In addition, my doctor urges me to supplement my daily diet with compressed greens that supply a healthy dose of chlorophyll.

The second example, which dates back to the late '80s when I ran a café in South America, had immediate tangible results. Despite my proactive and creative marketing and public relations tactics, sales were sluggish. While I loved the venue we chose and built for our business, a queasiness deep inside never left me. I felt bad vibes lingering. According to the rumor mill, our spot was once the scene of a violent crime.

Before we learned about the history, my husband said our rented space was *salado*, similar to being cursed. Our locale needed a limpia. We could have burned sulfur or copal and said prayers, but I had faith that a spiritual cleansing would be more forceful and sincere if an older family friend led the ritual.

Indigenous practices were second nature to Rosa, the woman who led the cleanses at our café. The day after one of her spiritual cleanings, our restaurant had record-breaking sales. I had to run to the market to get more cooking supplies.

Since that experience, I smudge my house periodically by burning small wrapped bundles of palo santo or sage. I try to channel the spirit of Rosa or others from whom I have learned these sacred traditions.

When I put my house on the market, I performed periodic smudges, recognizing that negative energy from potential homebuyers could enter any day. Then when I bought my new property, I smudged on closing day. I didn't just light a match and enjoy the smell. I repeated heartfelt prayers filled with positive visualizations as I cleansed the space with the smoke.

While smudging is both an Indigenous and East Indian tradition, today, the ritual is commonplace. Sage and palo santo are sold everywhere. During the pandemic, I smudged more frequently, believing in its scientific merit and hoping the smoke might protect against the COVID-19 virus.

In 2008, the Journal of Pharmacology published a study about medicinal smoke, a type of smoke generated by burning various natural substances, such as plants, incense and resins, for the purpose of therapeutic healing and purification of the environment. (Smudging is a more commonly known form of medicinal smoke.) Microbiologists at the National Botanical Research Institute in India[128] sought to substantiate the fire-burning practices described in the oldest of the sacred Hindu texts, the Rig Veda. They concluded that medicinal smoke reduces airborne bacteria by 94 percent. The study was based on a mix of dozens of herbs common to India.

One experiment found inhaling burning frankincense alleviated depression and anxiety.[129] Interestingly enough, this resin was sacred in Jerusalem during the time of Jesus and his disciples.

The wisdom and practices of the sages endured across continents, religions and time. These customs may have been somewhat dormant in our society, but people are returning to them. They give a sense of well-being and connection to the universe. Regardless of one's religion or lack of one, traditions such as Gloria's are both grounding and uplifting.

Give It a Try:
Prepare Blessed Moon Water

You can perform this ritual in just a few minutes every night or on special occasions when you feel you need extra prayers or strength. It doesn't matter if you can see the moon in the sky, but be aware that the effects will be most powerful during a full moon.

1. Get ready.
   Find a glass mason jar or a ceramic bowl. Fill the container with regular tap water.

2. Enjoy the invocations.
   Recite whatever is in your heart or your thoughts

at the moment. Pray at your altar, with or without candles. The following is an example of one of Gloria's spontaneous recitations.

"Let's pray and hope that this time of strife will soon pass. Let's pray we are ready to accept the newness ahead. All who have faith, together we can make magic and make it happen. Envision. Envision. Envision."

3. **Find a location.**

    At sundown, place the water outside in a safe place, out of reach of any pets, stray animals or passing people. For those who live in an apartment or if temperatures are below freezing outside, place the jar inside on a windowsill that faces the moonlight.

4. **Let the moon work on the water.**

    Bathe the water in the moonlight from sundown until you wake up.

5. **Bask in the water each time you reach for it.**

    In the morning, place your blessed water in your sacred space. Incorporate the water into your daily routine. For example, say a prayer as you pour drops into your tea or into your bath. Bask. Enjoy. Share.

Gloria freely contributes her spiritual traditions as a gift to her community, expecting nothing in return. There is a great benefit to selfless service, as we'll learn next.

Chapter 10: Serving is the Secret of Abundance

Service comes first. We gain more
from giving than from taking.

—Swami Sitaramananda

M y mom taught me it is better to give than to receive. My grandparents were immigrants who arrived at Ellis Island with nothing but open hearts and minds. For many years, my maternal grandparents lived in a tiny rural town set along a railroad track. My grandmother served meals to every hobo that knocked on her door. We called her actions by the Hebrew name *tzedakah*, the moral obligation to give to others.

Swami Sitaramananda, director of the Sivananda Yoga Farm in California and the Sivananda Yoga Resort and Training Center in Vietnam, encourages a similar principle of selfless service. In Swami Sita's tradition, it's called "karma yoga." Others call it by its Sanskrit name *seva*.

I shored up my commitment to selfless service after spending time with Swami Sita at the Yoga Farm. This spiritual master's teachings inspired me to make space for karma yoga, or my own acts of service, just as some people make space for a daily or weekly hatha yoga class. Lessons learned from her morning and evening chats are evident in my lifestyle today. The swami's words transformed my moral compass and jostled faulty patterns.

By 2010, I had been practicing yoga for more than thirty years when I hankered for more. I searched the internet for advanced training. The majority of offerings I found were too resort-y, too pricey, or too sham-y for me.

Despite the long plane, train and bus ride required to get to Grass Valley, California, Sivananda Yoga Farm was perfect. The Yoga Farm is an oasis for wholesomeness and nourishment in a pristine, austere environment. This spiritual, nonsectarian, nonprofit center for learning spreads over eighty peaceful, pollution-free wooded acres in the Sierra Nevada foothills. You are here and nowhere else. Isolated from urban sprawl, you cannot run to a gas station to feed your fix of coffee, beef jerky, soda or beer. (All items that are not allowed at the ashram.) One of the beauties about being at the Yoga Farm is its camp-like setting with wooden cabins, meals at picnic benches, and yoga outdoors.

The website was very explicit about the daily regimen. Wake up at 5:30 a.m. Meditate at 6 a.m. followed by a chat with Swami Sita. Enjoy two-hour yoga sessions before both lunch and dinner. Perform karma yoga work activities. Eat two *sattvic* (no caffeine, alcohol, meat or egg) meals a day. Chant in the evening, then attend another brief lecture by Swami Sita or a special guest speaker. Finally, turn the lights out at 10 p.m.

This ten-day experience was a holistic battery recharger for me. So much so that later I returned to the unpretentious ashram in the forest for nearly a month. My second Yoga Farm stay produced multiple positive behavioral shifts, as well as a boost to my self-esteem. One of the staff suggested I register for teacher training. Until that time, I hadn't seen myself as teacher material since I was not slim and trim, I was not young and pretty, and I most certainly did not wear Lycra.

The Sivananda way[130] has no typecast molds. Sivananda teachers represent all ages, all shapes, all ethnicities, and wear uniform short-sleeve T-shirts with loose-fitting cotton pants. The nonjudgmental, positive attitudes I felt at the Sivananda Yoga Farm gave me the confidence and inspiration to become a yoga teacher.

In addition, my foundation in Sivananda yoga whetted my appetite to learn more about the ancient Indian traditions. I soon dedicated myself to study Ayurveda at a Sivananda center in India. That training influenced me to pursue formal yoga therapy training. So, in reality, my first Sivananda intensive under the direction of Swami Sita completely transformed my life.

The Social Worker Yogi: Swami Sitaramananda

Swami Sita's transformation began when she was a young adult. She spent the first eighteen years of her life in Vietnam. In 1971, she flew west for graduate studies at the French-speaking University of Montreal. She wanted to help others. Without having heard the term "karma yoga," she entered into that discipline as a community organizer and social worker, but she burned out early.

> I always have been a karma yogi. One needs to change oneself before attempting to help the world. I realized yoga could give me a tool to make myself strong so I can help the world.

This twenty-eight-year-old social worker began her spiritual journey and reinforced her karma yogi instincts when she met her teacher from Swami Sivananda's lineage in Quebec.[131]

Impressed and intrigued by the Sivananda organization's messages and approaches, she worked for the nonprofit in Canada for a few years. Then, in 1985, she took a vow to commit her life to the higher good. She chose the path of a renunciate monastic yogi, dressed in saffron-colored robes, and with hair cropped to an inch or two. Some years later, she was sent to lead the Sivananda center in San Francisco before making the Yoga Farm her home base in 1995.

> Basically, I dedicated my life to teach yoga and help people, at the same time as living the yoga life.
> And that didn't burn me out [like social work did].
> It gave me a lot of energy.

In fact, the spiritual life gave her enough vigor to get by on a scant three or four hours of sleep a night. After disconnecting from her long day of karma yoga duties, her nighttime self-imposed work began: cramming to improve her command of the English language. I can picture the Swami's cheeky grin as she admits in her impeccable, but accented English, "You're not supposed to stay up late. So I didn't tell anyone."

With a schedule like that, it was difficult for her to incorporate her essential daily hatha physical yoga practice. But she managed to squeeze in her personal routine that includes breathwork and bodywork. Without it, she says she doesn't have the power to get through the day.

> It's an intense life. But the most beautiful, very inspired life, when you do things for a higher purpose: serving the mission of yoga. We are far more than our ego.

Swami Sivananda had the foresight [to see] that the West needed yoga. His motto was "Serve, love, give, purify, meditate, realize."

These six words are very important, but service comes first.

Each word in Swami Sivananda's motto is an element of yoga. But many are unaware of, or not interested in, the breadth and depth of yoga. They stop at the physical practice.

The Guru's Wisdom: Serve to Fuel the Spirit

Swami Sita says it is essential to go deeper. Understanding karma and karma yoga is like learning your ABCs. They are building blocks to healthy, happy and holistic living.

Swami Sita focused on the true essence of karma yoga during a global, virtual lecture from Vietnam, from which excerpts follow.[132] The online session featured simultaneous translations in Korean, Chinese, Russian and Japanese to impart the meaning and benefits of karma and karma yoga to her global community.

While karma may be a common word nowadays, more often than not, it is used without the proper context. A literal translation of the word "karma" is "action." But with every action, there is a reaction—cause and effect. However, consequences are not necessarily immediate as they are when you spill spaghetti sauce on a white shirt. The reaction can drag on, even into another lifetime.

Karma is like a wheel. What goes around, comes around. Let's say you break your leg. That action must have come from some other action in the past. Anything that happens has a reason.

Everyone has [baggage]. Karma manifests in many ways. There are thousands of combinations of different karmic situations. Some people are born as a prince... and some people are born with no support or are given away.

Your peace of mind is also part of your karma. When you have weaknesses, you create enemies, debts or diseases. Some people have the karma in life to have difficult relationships.

Looking for happiness is like running after your own shadow. Our culture and media fabricate unreal desires for storybook endings. Girls want to find Prince Charming or their bachelor in paradise. Many are after the pot of gold or the lottery jackpot. People tend to be busy running around in circles. The pursuit of happiness is futile. The only solution is to slow down and be wise in one's actions.

Some people want to be famous, and they never can be. You make money and lose money. It is not necessarily good or bad. It's just what people have to go through—and learn.

On the other hand, karma yoga is all about volunteering your time in service through thoughts, words and deeds.

Swami Sita gives a personal example to underscore how elusive true selfless service can be. After working around the clock serving hundreds of people for twenty years, Swami Sita finally got a break—real solitude and inaction. She found the answer in a cave in India, where she spent two months to withdraw and go within.

When you're very quiet and by yourself, there's a lot happening. It was wonderful. A time to contemplate.

I learned during that time that I wasn't a very good karma yogi.

Her breakthrough realization was that selflessness has no end and that she could do better with her selfless service. Despite all her benevolent deeds and pure intentions, she had not perfected the essence of karma yoga. It is not about the amount of money you donate or the number of hours you volunteer. It is all about your motive.

Swami Sita admires Mother Teresa. The short-statured Nobel Peace Prize winner never took credit for her monumental efforts. In her book, *The Joy of Living*, Saint Teresa wrote:

I am a little pencil in God's hands. He does the thinking. He does the writing. He does everything and sometimes it is really hard because it is a broken pencil and He has to sharpen it a little more.

That's the ideal attitude for a karma yogi.

Swami Sita points to Swami Sivananda as another true karma yogi. In addition to his devotion to yoga, he was a selfless medical doctor who treated people for free in Malaysia and India. Similar to Mother Teresa's words about function without attachment, he said, "I am only the instrument. It's not about me. I am here to serve."

According to Swami Sita:

There is no job higher or lower in karma yoga. Everyone's job is important. Just like all the organs of the body are necessary. See the big picture. Do your duty. If you wash the dishes, wash the dishes well. Do it with good spirit, not expecting anything [in return]. Be joyful, rather than scheming.

Sometimes, it is easier said than done. Swami Sita broke through spiritual roadblocks. At one point, she did chores that her ego did not appreciate. She washed people's clothes and served meals to students. Yet through those roles, she learned a fundamental lesson.

When the ego is in high gear, it leads to suffering. On the other hand, detachment leads to happiness. Remove the "I" from the equation. Thoughts should not be about what *I* like, what *I* want, what *I* need, or what *I* expect.

She notes:

> Desires are insatiable. When you can think of others and really give to others, your heart opens and the energy of the universe can flow through you. And you feel so good.

Another principle of karma yoga is to act without being fixated on the results. A doctor does the best he or she can but cannot cure everyone. Again, it is about the intent and the motive behind the action. It's natural for people to focus on a result, but what's important is to have a noble intention and to remove one's ego from the equation.

The swami refers to actions as deposits in your karmic bank account. Selfless actions, introspection, contemplative study, and meditation are all credits to counteract any negative activity.

> If you don't make an effort to pay your debt, you sink deeper into debt. If you don't make efforts to be wise, you sink deeper into ignorance. Anything you do that makes you wake up from your ignorance is credit. Anything that makes you more ignorant or egoistic is debt. So choose your action.

Practice karma yoga anytime, anywhere, with anybody. It's a convenient and practical path of breaking through the ego and finding yourself through selflessness.

In life, sometimes it's difficult to make choices. It's never perfect. Do the best you can.

Even though selfless service is not about getting anything in return, most of us feel a sense of satisfaction.

Yoga teaches us we are far more than our ego and the stories we assemble about who we are and what we like or don't like. It teaches that we are happier when we move out of our egoism and away from these thoughts to serve others, regardless of whether the mind likes it at first.

Through this service, one experiences an expansion of his or her sense of self.[133]

Swami Sita's Five Easy Tips

1. **Keep doing good acts.**

   Practice simple selfless service every day. It can be as simple as calling a sick friend or offering to pick up groceries for an elderly neighbor. As you do good things, know that as you raise your consciousness, you are helping the world.

2. **Be present.**

   Be aware. Don't focus on the past or the future. Be in the now and you will have fewer worries.

3. **Be happy.**

   Enjoy the selfless work you are doing. Do not react or lament. Your mind, body and spirit will appreciate it.

4. Keep calm.

Train yourself to slow down and be more mindful in all your actions, big or small.

5. Do the best you can. Surrender. Let go of expectations and results to practice true karma yoga.

Selfless Service for the Spirit

It feels so good to engage in service for others. It is challenging to shut out that sense of gratification, but Swami Sita says to let go of results. Disconnect the action from the reaction of feeling good or making people happy.

Society teaches us from the time we can walk to focus on the selfish finish line, the egoistic goal, the individual score, and the applause. We compare each other and have rankings, price tags and ratings for everything. It's hard to break free from the mentality built into one's culture.

During my selfless service experiences at Yoga Farm, I never felt judged. We all helped out as a team, and someone responsible for the kitchen or the groundskeeping guided us in our tasks. I enjoyed being active, not expecting any rewards. Usually, I washed dishes. Sometimes I helped with meal prep or gardening. There was an air of everyone pitching in, regardless of our duties and abilities.

On the other hand, I had a very unpleasant experience one year volunteering in Mexico. I heard about a young American couple looking for volunteers to join them at an orphanage in Mexico. Filled with a yearning to help the little children, I committed to come for a month. As a Spanish-speaker with experience teaching kids of all ages both yoga and English as a second language, I had great expectations. I wasn't alone.

Several of us had high hopes of sharing our diverse teaching skills at an orphanage. Our expectations led to overpowering frustrations. We could not disconnect our service from the inadequate management, lack of accountability, and potential dangers for the little ones. We found fault in processes and apparent disregard for the children. It was hard for us not to judge the people who lured us there or the nuns who ignored the kids. We followed our own initiatives to lead fun learning sessions. But that didn't go over well with the organizers. They booted us out one day, telling us to remove all our belongings and vacate the premises. To make it worse, they evicted us from the orphanage in front of the confused children, who were in our laps or hugging us.

In hindsight, considering the mission for which we signed up, we should have done our best with a smile and kind words rather than assign blame or hang on to expectations. We allowed our egos to interfere. We had better intentions than they did. We had more training than they did. We had better communication skills than they did. We had greater rapport with the kids than they did. That was a perfect example of when one's actions may be well intended but a need for self-fulfillment got in our way.

More recently, I spent a month volunteering as a yoga instructor in Nicaragua. This time, there were no expectations.

Aside from the yoga duties, the owner tasked me with another challenging, but important, role. I never said, "that's not why I'm here" or "that's not my forte." Rather, I trusted his judgment and was content to fill whatever void he felt was appropriate. I thrived in that setting and returned the next year for longer.

In 2022, I signed up to be a karma yogi for a month at an ashram in Italy. My job duties were not what I had hoped for, but it didn't matter. There was a beautiful spirit among all the other volunteers as we pulled weeds, swept floors, removed cobwebs, scrubbed bathrooms, or polished museum-grade picture frames.

One day, working in the kitchen, the head chef and I prepared lasagna for three hundred fifty people. I filled dozens of trays with layer after layer of oversized noodles, tomato sauce and cheese. In Italian, I confessed, I felt as if I should pay for this incredible opportunity to serve.

There has been plenty of research conducted around selfless service from the East and the West.

A 2013 study from India pointed to the emotional benefits of karma yoga, among them were enhanced satisfaction with life, reduced anxiety and apprehension, and even physical well-being.[134]

In 2022, researchers in Mumbai, India, evaluated karma yoga in the workplace. They noted a direct relationship between the level of service and mindfulness. Moreover, the analysis found that karma yoga contributed to a greater sense of "flourishing" or "thriving" in the workplace, while reducing burnout.[135]

In the West, Penn State psychology professor, John A. Johnson, PhD, wrote about karma yoga in a two-part series on selfless service for *Psychology Today* in 2013.[136] These articles include a laundry list of reasons karma yoga works and acknowledge a common hurdle—not expecting anything in return. Unconsciously, we relish even a smile or a thank you.

> Indeed, research indicates numerous benefits to those who engage in selfless service, including

reduction of emotional disturbance, greater longevity, stress reduction, improved morale, increased self-confidence and self-esteem, better health and pain reduction, and greater overall happiness.

When we help others without thought of personal gain, we can actually gain a lot...

Think about some of the humanitarian or volunteer efforts you've been involved with in the past, regardless of how simple or involved they may have been. Do you recall what your primary motivations were? How did you feel about helping?

I suspect Jimmy and Rosalynn Carter have invested hundreds of hours building houses for the poor simply for humanitarian reasons. While most of us are probably not as selfless as the Carters, Swami Sita encourages people to "just do your best."

||||||||||||||||||||||||||||||||||||||||||||||||||||||||||||||||||||||||||||||||||||||||||||||||||||||||||||||||||||||||||||||||||||||||

Give It a Try:
Make a Date to Be Selfless

There are so many ways in which one can practice selfless service. If you are already a part of a faith- or community-based organization, offer to help where the need is greatest.

Rather than saying "I like to cook—I'll volunteer in the kitchen," ask "Where is the greatest need for my time?"

Most cities have an endless list of charitable organizations that are lacking human resources. Whether it is doing manual labor, accounting, translations or providing companionship, all services are important. Have an open mind and an open heart with a smile on your face, regardless of what your assignment is.

There are also many ways to volunteer your time, skills or monetary donations without ever leaving your home. When you want to buy any product, see if you can purchase it from a nonprofit or small business rather than a mass-retailer.

When you get the travel bug, consider voluntourism, where options abound. Some of my greatest travel experiences have been as a volunteer in Nicaragua and Italy.

Don't limit your Thanksgiving to one Thursday a year. Give thanks year-round. Give of your time, money, energy, wisdom and creativity without expecting anything in return. And instill the same desire in your children.

The next guru not only exemplifies the meaning of a karma yogi, but he enlists an inordinate number of people around the world (including me) to render service to the underserved.

Chapter 11: Happiness Isn't a Big Bank Account

We lose ourselves [...] with materialism.
We're obsessed with the things money can buy.

—Radhanath Swami

For a kid from the Chicago suburbs, Radhanath Swami followed a nontraditional life as part of his journey within. Today, leading thousands in spiritual and social enterprises from his ashram in Mumbai, India, the gracious guru meets with leaders around the world. He is a primary force behind a charity hospital, mobile eye and dental camps, and a program that feeds three hundred thousand people daily. He is at the helm of an award-winning ecovillage, a women's empowerment initiative, and several financial literacy programs.

As an ascetic, His Holiness Radhanath Swami lives an austere life. He closed his meager bank account fifty years ago and now travels around the world with no possessions. His wealth comes from his spirituality, not the material world.

I first encountered this unassuming swami at a retreat in the 100°F heat of the Southern California desert. He was not preachy. He was funny, like the guy next door, only wearing an orange robe with a shaven head and carrying prayer beads. While he is not a musician, he led the most tender kirtan that would amp into ecstatic song and dance with more than one hundred people jumping up and down with joyous energy.

I returned to that scene annually when Radhanath Swami toured the States, squeezing in among the crowds of primarily youthful Californians that welcomed him like a saint. Every time I was in the presence of the humble spiritual leader, I took notes or recorded his talks that were chock-full of wisdom.

Even though there were hundreds in the audience, seated on the floor with knees and shoulders bumping into one another, I always found my way to the front. Up close, I could better catch the expressions on the swami's face as he recounted hilarious tales of his parents visiting him in India, the scary parts of his life journey, and the holiest ones too.

Not far from where both he and I were raised, I attended several of his chats in more intimate settings. Seated an arm's length away, I exchanged a few words with him, and on two occasions, his childhood friend took photos of us together.

The most heartfelt of all my encounters was when I was on his home turf in India. With a majestic sandstone and marble temple in South Mumbai as a backdrop, the revered spiritual master envisioned and oversaw a flower festival representing the beauty in diversity that drew thousands of participants. Radhanath Swami helped build and transform what was once a meager room into a sizable complex for prayer, work, study and dorm spaces modeled after seventeen temples in the holy city of Vrindavan, India.

The majority of people who attended in person viewed the elaborate event from monitors on the temple patio, while others from around the world tuned in to the livestream. I was among a few dozen seated near the swami. The ceremony felt as big as New Year's Eve in New York City's Times Square, but it was a celebration radiating spirituality, joy and respect for all beings.

During that trip, the spiritual master invited my small group into his library to welcome us to India and answer questions. Copies of his memoir, translated to more than twenty languages, filled the walls, like wallpaper lining the room.

The next day, my fellow travelers and I left the overcrowded pollution-filled Mumbai megalopolis to visit Govardhan Ecovillage. It is a planned, sustainable community, a few hours north of Mumbai. The wellness and retreat center, Radhanath Swami's brainchild, is the recipient of more than twenty-five awards, including the Award for Excellence and Innovation in Tourism from the United Nations World Tourism Organization.

Govardhan Ecovillage is a stark contrast to urban India. At the retreat center, we gathered around Radhanath Swami, sitting cross-legged on cow-patty floors, to sing and hear his stories. The ambiance was reminiscent of peaceful summer campfires when the surroundings, camaraderie and activities are blissful.

The Indiana Jones of Spiritual Seekers: Radhanath Swami

The story of how the kid from Chicago, Richard Slavin, ended up as His Holiness Radhanath Swami is retold in his bestselling memoir, The Journey Home, which reads like a cross between The Little Buddha and Indiana Jones and the Raiders of the Lost Ark. His tale proves life is stranger than fiction as he recounts his journey, leaving the comforts of suburbia to go hungry and sleep in caves and under trees searching for true happiness. "I was homeless, but felt so much at home," he recounts of his early days in India.

Richard went to a top-ranked, predominantly White public high school during the time of the Vietnam War. Pretty much all his classmates were college-bound, but Richard was not like the rest.

His father went bankrupt, and money was tight. For extra income, Richard worked at a car wash with minority kids from lower socioeconomic families, which heightened his sensitivity to the plight of people of color.

> They all had no way out. I really loved them. I remember thinking, "Why is it they have no opportunities?" A lot of things didn't make sense to me.

It was a time of turmoil. The assassinations of Rev. Dr. Martin Luther King, Jr., and President John F. Kennedy, both of whom fought for social justice and equality, were a major blow to this idealistic kid from a privileged community.

Young Richard chose to be part of the change. He let his hair grow long. He sported a straggly beard and mustache, dressed in faded jeans and a black vest, and identified with the counterculture. With a grin, he shares:

> I ended up [demonstrating for civil rights] at Grant Park during the Democratic convention. And I am proud to say I got tear-gassed by the Chicago Police.

After his first year of college, he joined two pals in Europe for summer break, one of whom offered to pick up much of the cost. Almost as soon as they arrived, the kid with the dough got pickpocketed. Without his credit cards and cash, the friend jumped on a return flight back to Chicago. Richard and Gary stayed. With only twenty dollars in his pocket, Richard and his best friend chose to rough it. They hitchhiked from one bare-bones hostel to another and from one hippie festival to the next, where they could find free food and a place to sleep.

At one point in the United Kingdom, judging them to be penniless druggies, the "bobbies" interrogated them for an hour and threatened to cut off their long hair.

Richard began an intense quest to find himself and the meaning of the universe. He recalls:

> In my heart, there were serious questions I had to address in my life. I concluded that real solutions have to be found within one's self. I started doing some yoga and meditation and read different scriptures.

Perched on a remote mountaintop in Greece, he and Gary meditated. When they reopened their eyes, they were each jubilant. A spark of wisdom flashed in their respective silent reflective moments. They each received seminal messages and were elated to share their respective visions. Gary's inspiration directed him to find answers in Israel. Richard had a similar revelation, but his destination was India.

The best friends said their farewells as they followed their destinies to different holy lands.

Richard had no money—not even for bus or train fare. The journey to his promised land meant traversing 4,000 miles through seven countries, several of which were war-torn. His prized possession fit in his pocket: a harmonica.

It took Richard six months, bumming rides and walking, to get from the Greek island mountaintop to Lahore at the southern edge of Pakistan.

Reflecting on his long trek, he notes that most people would choose a comfortable eight hours of flight time on British Airways. "But it's not as scenic or life-changing," he laughs.

Catching glimpses of India on the other side of the border, the dust-covered, emaciated boy with grand dreams thought he was in heaven. In reality, he was in limbo. The border patrol would not allow him to cross. He was in a desolate area, and there was an ongoing conflict between Pakistan and India. To make matters worse, his visible assets consisted of twenty-six cents in five currencies.

The border agent told him, "We have enough beggars in India. We don't want another one."

He pleaded with no luck and found a tree to take shelter. After six hours, he begged again. The response was even worse. "They put their guns in my face and said, 'If you come back we will kill you.'"

When there was a change in guards, he gave it another try. He promised a Sikh border patrolman that he would improve the lives of the people of India someday. With Richard's sickly beggar-like appearance at the time, it is hard to imagine that a compassionate guard had faith in those claims and would let him cross. It was improbable that one day Radhanath Swami would contribute to the well-being and transformation of India through many charitable, educational and spiritual enterprises. Yet something made the guard let Richard pass anyway.

His spiritual journey was not smooth sailing once he crossed the border. He found that there is no litmus test for gurus. Richard knew the real gurus would be sages to lead one from darkness into light, from ignorance to knowledge, and from suffering to true happiness. But what he encountered were many false gurus who offered empty promises and claimed to be what they were not.

When he reached the holy town of Vrindavan, 100 miles south of Delhi, Richard chanced upon Srila Prabhupada,[137] the founder of the International Society for Krishna Consciousness, who advocated the yogic path of bhakti.

I met so many gurus who had so many philosophies. In 1971, I was among five or six other people sitting around Srila Prabhupada. He wasn't my guru then. He was just one of the [many] saints I was coming to visit.

Somebody asked him, "Are you the guru for the whole world?"

He didn't respond. Most people would say, "Yes." Instead, he paused for a few minutes, looking at the ground. With tears of humility in his eyes, he said, "No, I am the servant of everyone. That's all."

A true guru is not one who claims to be God. A true guru is one who claims to be a humble messenger of God.

At last, Richard had found a place he never wanted to leave and a spiritual guide he admired. But roadblocks remained. Engrossed in his spiritual learning, he ignored the details of his entry permit. With an expired visa, the serene young man who was entrenched in the divine was now a fugitive with an immigration agent out to catch him.

The solution to his expired visa was beyond anyone's imagination. It was not a bribe or leaving the country.

A rabid animal pulled him into a sewer and infected him with rabies. While the urgent medical treatment is a nightmare to most, it resulted in the government granting him an emergency visa.

Ultimately, he remained in India for several more years before his first visit back to the States, which he laughingly admits was not the best timing. George Harrison and Ravi Shankar stayed at his ashram just a few days after he left.

It's safe to say his parents were a little surprised when they greeted a different son two years later at the airport. Richard was not the same college kid who had left home to have fun in Europe. He was now an ascetic following an ancient spiritual path. He had no suitcases, backpacks or duffel bags—only a beggar's pot, prayer beads and a small cotton bag.

The Guru's Wisdom: Treasure True Gifts

"In all the great spiritual traditions, the real wealth is in our state of mind." But Radhanath Swami cautions, "When you expect things, you are never happy." Whether we have a lot of possessions or a little is irrelevant. It doesn't matter whether one is a surgeon or a garbage man. We are all created in God's image, and we are all equal.

Radhanath Swami believes we own nothing. Everything, even the organs in our body, are gifts from the Creator and belong to the universe. Likewise, the same God is in all of us. Humanity is a sisterhood and brotherhood unfolding from the same source.

> One sees a child of God wherever there is life. And one respects, one honors, one loves that living force within nature—the plants and trees, the birds, animals and all varieties of human beings.

In our society, we tend to create measurements of scale and seek to rise to the top. Yet if we all come from the same source, then no one human is better than another and no one species is higher than the next.

A person's greatness is not measured by wealth, land, beauty or athletic ability. Rather, greatness is measured by how we respond to challenging situations.

> What is true greatness? It's humbling oneself to the infinite grace of the Supreme. When we connect with the love of God, we find even greater joy in seeing the success of others.

We should not let the ego get in the way. Rather, we should act with a higher purpose for the good of others, society and our world.

> We always have free will—whether in pleasant times or in hard times. We can make choices to live with integrity. This is what life is about.

> But how many things in the universe can we *not* control? Limitless. That should humble us.

Life is like ripples in a pond. One movement or action leads to corresponding waves.

> Every choice we make affects our destiny. You can tell how rich you are by counting [what] you have that money *cannot* buy. Peace. Love. These things bring purpose to life. *Things* can never give fulfillment to the heart.

> When I was a boy, for my mother's birthday, I would steal a flower from her garden, and she would cry from happiness. It's the thought of love that gives value.

An expression of sincere love and kindness, regardless of the price tag, is meaningful and memorable.

Humans were not born with huge closets, basements or storage units to house an infinite number of material items. Cave dwellers stockpiled food just to tide them over during the winters. We are not hardwired to accumulate objects but to love and to be loved. That is why selfless love for all beings is the greatest gift we can pass on to our children.

> In the heart that harbors the weed of selfish greed, the flower of love cannot survive. Love is inherent within everyone. It is our essence. Our nature is to love. Appreciation is an expression of love. People thrive when they are appreciated. It doesn't cost anything, but it can bring great fulfillment. And what greater opportunity is there than to recognize this and prioritize and seek this in times of turbulence?

To love means to serve. While the intent is to uplift others, there is no greater joy than selfless service. It is better to give than to receive.

Radhanath Swami recounts the story of an American surgeon volunteering for one of his organization's sliding-scale hospitals in India. The doctor tended to a cheerful, disabled boy, toiling for hours in the operating room to realign the youngster's limbs. After the surgery, the convalescing patient lavished the practitioner with appreciation for helping to cure him of his state. Endearingly, the child said, "Doctor, you are a wonderful person."

Those words meant the world to the surgeon. "I do surgery on VIPs and they pay me a fortune, but I've never been so happy as with the words of appreciation from this child," he noted.

In another case, His Holiness spoke of one of his medical missions to restore vision to the sightless. The volunteer doctors work twelve hours a day to treat three thousand people within one month. The patients, dressed in rags, are so impoverished that they cherish even a drop of water. Many are emaciated, and few have ever seen a doctor before.

While most of us take it for granted that eyeglasses, contact lenses, laser treatment or LASIK surgery will improve our visual clarity, these villagers only anticipate blindness. In the case of one elderly woman treated at the ISKCON eye camp, when the bandages were removed, she was ecstatic. For the first time in years, she could see peoples' faces. She overwhelmed the doctor with her joy, praise and appreciation.

Radhanath Swami reflected:

> That lady was wealthy with a love of God and blessings. Real wealth is to love and be loved, between *atma* (the eternal soul) and God or whatever you may call him. When we open our hearts, we become full of happiness and instruments of love. Love empowers us.

Modern society encourages focusing on the material rather than our spirit, intellect, loving-kindness or respect for other sentient beings and our planet. Referring to materialism, Radhanath Swami says, "We are being bombarded by weapons of mass destruction." Not everything man creates is good. But if man attempts to be an instrument of God's love, we can grow rather than destroy.

There is boundless intelligence in nature. Radhanath Swami recounts when he was in Bahrain in the Persian Gulf, he chanced upon a miracle in a no man's land. Amid an endless sea of scorching sand and stifling 120°F dusty air, there was a green spot.

> We drove into a desert where there was no life to be seen anywhere. And in this desert, there was a tree—a huge tree, full of green leaves. It's been there for a hundred years. They call it the "tree of life." Somehow, where there are sandstorms and heat storms, that tree keeps growing. And in doing so, it shows us how we can grow in difficult circumstances. Many of the greatest advances in science, technology or sports have come in times of great crisis.

Conversely, serious problems arise from shallow perspectives when people focus on the exterior or the superficial, like the car, house or watch.

> The deeper and more inclusive our awareness is, the more we can find joy and share it. When we connect to that inner self, we understand our true harmony with God and with all human beings, life and nature. We're no longer finding joy in exploiting. We become instruments of compassion. When we connect to our true self, that's when the spiritual dimension of our life unfolds. And that's where the greatest meaning and purpose can be [found]. When we forget the treasures within us, we struggle to find happiness through this body and mind.

It is possible to find happiness that outshines the biggest diamond.

Radhanath Swami sums it up.

Happiness is not in acquisition, but in inner realization. If we are not happy within, we cannot be happy under any circumstances.

Radhanath Swami's Five Easy Tips

1. Love, to attract love.

   True wealth is to love and be loved. Love life. Love yourself. Love humanity. Love other species. Love the planet.

2. Engage your God-given gifts with a mindset of gratitude in service to others.

   Your skills or assets are sacred gifts. Share them as a gift of love.

3. Earn with integrity and spend with compassion.

   Be active in the world, but stay rooted in the soil of honesty and grace. Every dollar you earn or spend can make a difference when done with integrity and care.

4. Recognize the higher power behind your success and share the credit with others.

   This will give you pure joy. Taking all the credit for an accomplishment may satisfy the ego but will deprive the heart.

5. Be a nonconformist.

   In today's world, we are often encouraged to love material things and use people. Do the reverse. Embrace the evolved spiritual culture of loving people and using things to facilitate that love.

Letting Go of Material Securities

Over the years, I have heard many accounts about the happiness of those in economically oppressed countries. There are many rankings of the happiest people in the world based on numerous factors. While it is hard to score people's happiness levels based on their smiles, my experience mirrors what Radhanath Swami teaches. True happiness is not dependent upon economic success.

Having lived and spent extended periods in several developing nations, I agree that loving relations and communities are worth their weight in gold. The level of comfort from friends, families and neighbors generates a deeper sense of gratification or contentment[138] than a large house with a security gate can provide.

There is plenty of research that suggests the size of your bank deposits does not reflect your level of contentment.

A collaborative report between researchers at Harvard, the University of British Columbia, and the University of Virginia shows that money only goes so far in creating contentment and peace.[139] Based on empirical research the authors suggested consumers will feel better if they spend their money on experiences rather than material goods and donate to charitable causes.

A research review from Harvard Business School, the University of Mannheim in Germany, and BlackRock investment management company evaluated the happiness of millionaires.[140] The tipping point was bewildering. It took $8 million to make a difference in the level of happiness between those with less than $8 million and your average nonmillionaire.

The same team assessed contentment among lottery winners with prizes of several hundred thousand dollars. It seems the winning ticket was not a ticket to happiness. Instead, the winners were less likely to socialize than the average person and faced greater levels of mental stress.

A third analysis in the Harvard report was regarding the source of wealth. The self-made millionaires reported greater levels of satisfaction and joy compared to those who inherited their fortunes, indicating that our efforts and achievements contribute to happiness.

Materialism and the pleasure it provides are all relative. Humans are adaptable. Just as one person's junk is another's treasure, it all depends on what you become accustomed to. For the person in a mansion with five cars and servants, that sixth car means very little, whereas a free tank of gas can be a godsend to someone on a fixed income.

As Radhanath Swami says, "Whether we have everything or nothing, if we simply have devotion, we have everything."

In many communities, two-car garages and fenced-in yards are the norms. Inside, homes often have towering ceilings, walk-in closets, entertainment rooms with huge recliners, and giant plasma displays. It is not uncommon to rent air-conditioned storage units for belongings. The accumulation may be to fill other voids.

Comedian George Carlin got plenty of laughs when he said:

> A house is just a place to keep your stuff while you go out and get more stuff. That's the whole meaning of life—trying to find a place for your stuff.

Minimalist that I am, when I bought my new house, I loaded everything except one bed, a fridge, and a washer and dryer set into my Toyota Prius. It took several trips, but nothing was too large to squeeze inside my subcompact car.

The toughest part of moving from my home after twenty-one years was sorting through treasured photographs. These were my memories of fifty years of travel and hand-me-down family albums that chronicled ancestors in the old country. In the end, all my images fit in one cardboard box.

Harder than letting go of the material was leaving my job. In a way, the decision was spurred by the teachings of Radhanath Swami, who was the spiritual master of one of my teachers. My teacher's innocent remarks about morality and integrity fueled the fire of my discontent. For decades, I was a responsible breadwinner working around the clock for clients and services that did not jibe with my beliefs. Work boosted my ego and my pocketbook but trampled my spirit. I dreamed of using my talents in a positive way that meshed with my values and yearned to contribute to society.

My attachment to the workplace was not my coworkers or a need for mental stimulation, but the security of a steady income, employer-subsidized healthcare, and other company benefits. All my life, I depended on my paychecks. I was never unemployed for more than a month or two, even when moving to different countries or when my daughter was born.

I recognize that my attachments as a workaholic in constant fear of losing my job were unhealthy. Once I severed those ties, my spiritual life got a reboot, as did my physical and emotional well-being.

Give It a Try:
Say Goodbye to Some Possessions

In his autobiography, *The Journey Home*, Radhanath Swami speaks of his attachment to his beloved pocket-sized harmonica. It represented his trek from Europe to India and was the only item of value he kept. An inspirational moment in the book was when he tossed the instrument into the Ganges River as a renouncement of attachment to material goods. The reader feels the pain of giving up this one small pleasure. After a pang of grief for the lost harmonica, that emptiness is filled ten times over with newfound spirituality.

Many who ascribe to Radhanath Swami's teachings rid themselves of material items. Bestselling author and social media personality, Jay Shetty, spent three years as a monk in Radhanath Swami's ashram and sustainable village. Like the others, he gave up material comforts and slept on a thin mat on a hard floor. Spiritual bounty filled the void.

While it's safe to assume no one wants to be *possessed*, there is a tendency in our society to associate possessing material items with greatness. Fueled by the marketing world, which encourages consumers to consume, too often people use purchases as a form of therapy. However, too many possessions can drag us down. When we release material items, we tend to feel lighter, as highlighted in Marie Kondo's bestselling books *Spark Joy* and *The Life-Changing Magic of Tidying Up*.

To exercise a release from possessions, take a few days to purge whatever does not spark joy in your heart. Start with all your clothing. Then go to your books. Miscellaneous items should be sorted through later. Donate the items you rarely use to one of your favorite charities.

Imagine the joy someone less fortunate will take from items that are of limited worth to you. As you hand over your items, know that your donation is an act of love, gratitude and release, which has more value than anything else in life.

Downsizing material possessions doesn't mean erasing memories. After you say goodbye to your unnecessary items, be thankful for what you once had and all the nonmaterial blessings in your life. A sense of gratitude, as you'll see next, is indispensable.

Chapter 12: The Grace in Gratitude Is a Total Knockout

There is always something to be grateful for.
I carry zero negativities to bed with me.

—Brenda Bell

After living in San Antonio for twenty-one years, I moved to a quaint town in Texas Hill Country surrounded by beautiful wildflowers, enormous cypress trees, and winding creeks dotted with shale and sandstone rocks. I found a serene studio that combined Eastern martial arts with spiritual practices. I welcomed the opportunity to lead yin and yang balancing yoga in an environment where shoes were left by the front door, incense was always burning, and everyone bowed before entering the room. In my first conversation with the owner, a hapkido (Korean martial arts) master, he had glowing praise for his studio tai chi partner. Brenda Bell, he said, was a former high-ranking boxer. But more noteworthy, she had a radiant soul.

Brenda Bell, known as the "Tiger Lady," is the picture of gratitude and contentment, despite chronic pain, PTSD and dementia pugilistica. She overcame her physical, emotional and cognitive battles through the power of positivity.

Although I had dabbled in tai chi and respected the art and movement practice, I had never met a teacher like Brenda before. She was different. She attended my yoga classes, and I took part in her tai chi sessions. I felt the yogi in her. Whether she was the student or the teacher, she radiated a spiritual core and a soul full of gratitude. I wanted to catch her positive vibes.

Her teachings were a combination of tai chi, qi gong, and what she called "yoga in motion." I learned far more than the movements. She donned an impeccable, white, long-sleeved uniform that confirmed her respect for self and the practice.

Outside of the studio, where I felt like we were mind/body soul sisters, we collaborated elsewhere in my new community. I was a primary instructor for the "Livestrong at the YMCA" program, which provides cancer survivors throughout the United States with complementary holistic fitness classes. I looked forward to Brenda's guest lectures for our small close-knit groups, which changed members every twelve weeks.

I knew Brenda's story and coaching style were what my students needed. Under her direction, even the weak and infirm and those facing dismal prognoses could benefit from her flowing martial art form and heartfelt sense of appreciation for every moment lived.

Sporting close-cropped dark hair with a few curly gray strands at the temples and simple wire-framed glasses, she seemed to always stand at, and garner, attention. In perfect posture, she was ever ready for her tai chi moves, ready to fill her lungs with fresh air and to shine a broad smile to reflect immense gratitude.

Before, during and after every class, Brenda shared her mantra. "Yes! Yes! Yes! All is well." The soft-spoken instructor's infinite sense of gratitude and positivity were forceful. Each participant benefited from her characteristic display of appreciation and thanks for every day, every moment, every movement, and every breath.

Brenda's graceful, gentle practices, combined with her pep talks and positivity, were more than just martial arts. It may seem that tai chi and boxing are practices that are at odds. Knockouts conflict with peacefulness. Mercilessness is opposed to mindfulness. The drive to win seems unharmonious with the wisdom of surrender. But Brenda was able to balance those characteristics.

Sometimes life can be a bitch. According to many world philosophies, suffering is inescapable but can be overcome. Regardless of what troubles envelop you, you have the power to live a happy, healthy life. Gratitude can help you get there. Feel thankful for all life's blessings.

The Tiger Lady: Brenda Bell

The name "Brenda" means "flame" or "sword." All the weapons she carries now are imaginary. But at one time, those hands were encased in boxing gloves. Today her hands and feet stay bare. Her presentation of tai chi moves, like "Single Whip," "Carry Tiger," and "Repulse Monkey," are ancient, graceful, smooth-flowing defense forms passed on by generations of Chinese masters.

Her surname, Bell, evokes the harsh clang of the ringside bell that energized her to go out and win. Today, she moves like a bird in the wind to delicate sounds of Chinese panpipes, flutes, chimes and bamboo percussion.

Fresh out of high school, under the tutelage of a two-time karate Olympic champion, this peaceful soul earned her first *dan*, or black belt.

By twenty-three, at the pinnacle of her martial arts career, she began sparring. Brenda had unstoppable, steel-strength focus and discipline. She trained seven days a week. Sometimes, she was in the gym all day. There were never-ending rigorous diets and daily weigh-ins. That harsh drill was her new normal.

> Each day was made up of different regimens, which taught me new ways of knowing myself mentally and physically. My goal was to be the best in the world and fight the top women fighters of the world.

Wanting more challenges, her ambition steered her from Texas to California in 1987. She landed a job teaching tae kwon do in the Los Angeles area and became a student of a leading Korean martial arts master. She lived and breathed the philosophy, movements and meditations of that tradition.

A year later, she became one of an elite group of students residing within the martial arts studio. It was not a free ride by any means. She worked two jobs on the side to contribute to her training, room and board.

As she recalls:

> Everything was going according to my routine. As the highest-ranking female at the time, I lived and trained in the school. I wanted to improve myself and never doubted my ability. Setting my sights on being the best instructor out there, I continued to train despite criticism, stereotyping and setbacks.

That same year, she experienced the first of several assaults in Southern California. Dressed in her karate pants as she paid for gasoline, a man approached her and shoved a hard object into her side. For some odd reason, he ran off with Brenda's car keys—but not the car.

The second robbery was in a secluded, high-income neighborhood. Brenda was jogging with a heavy backpack when she was struck with a two-by-four in the head. As she fell to the ground, she saw four men surrounding her. They ran off with her backpack. The contents were not what the robbers expected: sandbags she used for endurance training.

While those acts of violence contributed to PTSD and chronic pain, she held no grudges toward the perpetrators. There were worse traumas yet to come.

In 1992, she was studying criminal justice at El Camino College, just twelve minutes south of Los Angeles International Airport. The reality of racial profiling, police brutality and inequities in the justice system set in. Four Los Angeles Police Department officers savagely beat Rodney King, an African American. The news media aired the videotaped attack for the world to see, yet a primarily White jury acquitted the attackers. Chaos in the city ensued. Los Angeles was in flames, and sixty-four people died.

Brenda, also an African American, was living in Hawthorne, California, with fellow martial arts trainees.

> The smell of smoke from the nearby riots was coming into our building. We made sure to watch the news to see what to do next to survive. It was scary for me, but I had to show my tough side.

Her instructor urged her to find safety outside the Hawthorne and Los Angeles area. She lived in her car for a week until the riots calmed down. She freshened up at a five-star hotel where she worked as a security guard.

> The safest place for me to go was the beach area, which kept me alive. PTSD had me. I couldn't shake things off. I would constantly turn around to see who was walking behind me. I wondered if I would get hit in the head again or if the person behind me might have a gun.

To the outside world, she was unflappable. Then one June early evening in 1994, the world watched as the Los Angeles Police Department chased O. J. Simpson for nearly an hour. Brenda was nearby. The shrill sound of the persistent sirens and watching the helicopters circling low in the air triggered her PTSD. Fear and anxiety permeated the martial arts champ and budding boxer. Despite her unsteady nerves brought on by the disorder, she continued to show her Rocky Balboa exterior.

Soon after, Brenda entered the professional boxing arena with the stage name of Tiger Lady. She shot up in the rankings.

In the year 2000, in Tunica, Mississippi, the Tiger Lady beat her competitor in a six-round unanimous decision. In the third round alone, Brenda came at her opponent with ninety-seven punches.

In November 2001, the Women's Boxing Archive Network named her "Fighter of the Month." The Tiger Lady was thirty-eight years old and past the prime for most boxers. Yet her jabs and uppercuts were still clobbering the top professionals in her weight class. The boxing network said, "Brenda truly represents the elite of guts, determination and fearlessness in women's boxing."

Brenda says:

> I was taught to work 70 percent mental and
> 30 percent physical. I kept my head up, knowing
> I was strong mentally. My personal growth had
> become a powerful goal that was more significant
> than material successes.

She was committed to being true to herself. At the same time, she was unrelenting because she shared Muhammad Ali's mentality: she could float like a butterfly and sting like a bee.

"I was at the top, knowing I was a match to the best fighters of the world," the Tiger Lady says.

Like Ali, too many injuries in the ring caused Brenda permanent brain damage. Boxers refer to the result as "punch drunk." But it doesn't wear off in the morning or with an aspirin. The official diagnosis, called "dementia pugilistica," causes cognitive impairment as well as speech, mood and behavioral disturbances. The serious irreversible condition frequently mimics parkinsonism.

Ultimately, the peaceful Tiger Lady's biggest fights were not in the ring, but with her brain. There is no reset button for dementia pugilistica. For a time, she fell into the depths of depression.

> I felt useless, beating myself up at the time. I had
> overwhelming concerns driving me too fast. I
> didn't know how to cancel my stupid ways. It
> was hard to let go. Sometimes I felt so sad that I
> thought I would never be happy again. Other
> times I was feeling almost nothing. As time went
> on, I knew God was at work in my life in ways that
> would strengthen my faith and wake me up with
> a solid purpose.

It was not just the brain injuries attacking her game plan. With one trauma after another, she officially retired from the ring in 2009.

Back home in Texas, she admitted herself into a residential brain center. After nine months, her cognitive behavior improved. But now she was overloaded with medications and had to readjust to society. As part of her depression and physical inactivity, she shot up from 150 to 400 pounds.

> I was giving up on my life. There was no reason for me to live. I was suicidal, and I was losing it. There were times I fell hard and was unable to get up because I had just lost hope.

But she kept in mind the Dalai Lama's words: "Happiness is not something ready-made. It comes from your own actions."

The Guru's Wisdom: Give Thanks

Today, Brenda recognizes she was mourning the life that had ended—her life as a prizefighter. Fortunately, her inherent positive winning attitude resurfaced and gave her the strength to overcome her toughest battles.

> All my life I have been positive, happy and loved to smile. Smiling brings me to a whole new level of life. I was born to win. Born for greatness... to be a champion in life.

She needed to accept her greatness outside the ring, so she fought her darkest moments head-on.

> I've come a long way to improve myself and to understand one thing that is important in my life today—to not miss out on opportunities, to come alive and feel more energetic.

She surrounded herself with sparks of positivity and kept her eye on the good in life. Brenda soaked up the words of one of the top motivational trainers, Brendon Burchard, author of *The Motivation Manifesto* and *Life's Golden Ticket*. His books gave her needed boosts to reignite her gratitude groove.

With the extra kick to thrive, Brenda returned to the comfort zone of the martial arts world—this time with her guru, Dr. Keith Jeffery, creator of Easy Tai Chi. The retired veterinarian, musician and motivational speaker combines East with West to accommodate modern-day folks living in a hectic world. Dr. Jeffery's style of tai chi and qi gong incorporates yogic principles of mindfulness with fluid body movement and breathwork.

The tai chi contributed to Brenda's cognitive functioning comeback. Plus, Easy Tai Chi reconnected Brenda to her body, mind and self-respect. As a result, she lost more than 200 pounds. Her happiness was reignited. Her can-do gratitude attitude came back as if on autopilot, spreading like wildfires to those around her.

> Dr. Jeffery's forms and meditations encourage me to go within, exploring myself first. Easy Tai Chi taught me to be softer and to show patience. It helped me beat my depression and anxiety—to be mindful. I learned what is true to me. That's when I know I am thankful. It's beautiful.

With no place for playing the victim, Brenda fills her mind, body and spirit with grace, gratitude and devotional music. Among her favorite recordings are Tina Turner's mantras. These are not like the supercharged rhythms of "Proud Mary" or "We Don't Need Another Hero." Brenda favors Tina's spiritual tunes. Among them is the sacred Sanskrit serenity prayer, "Sarvesham Svastir Bhavatu." One translation of it is:

> May there be happiness in all. May there be peace in all. May there be completeness in all. May there be success in all. Om. Peace. Peace. Peace.

Another favorite chant of Brenda's comes from Tina's *Beyond* album, "Sound of the Mystic Law: Lotus Sutra." The words in this Japanese Buddhist mantra are repeated at least 108 times, as the tradition calls for, to alleviate pain, suffering and bad karma.

Brenda says:

> I am still learning to live with the invincible physical pain I carry every day. But I feed myself with uplifting messages. Most important, I surround myself with people who keep my spirits up. I believe we all need to maintain a positive attitude and take care of ourselves for our own peace of mind. I stay in an upbeat mode every day.

Brenda teaches what she preaches. Several times a day, she leads groups of people from young fitness enthusiasts to seniors in nursing homes. One practice she shares is Dr. Jeffery's Four Minute Fitness tai chi program, which is broken into five components. Each element is a powerful repetition of either a mantra or an affirmation in movement. They include: Now is the only time, Love/Acceptance, Strength, Gratitude and All is Well. All components contribute to Brenda's essence of gratitude.

Her influence has not gone unnoticed. In 2021, the Original Warrior Association, a nonprofit member of the Black Karate Federation, honored her with a prestigious Grandmaster Belt for her dedication to martial arts and mentoring underprivileged children.

Today, with ever-present thanks, she is darn close to nailing her Chinese splits, the gymnastic middle straddle stretch that is tough even for young kids—no matter that she's not twenty-four any longer and is living with chronic pain. "I feel so right. I am able to smile," she says.

Her daily practice is filled with things to keep her positive. For example, some days, she reminds herself how thankful she is for each new day by jotting down things, big or small, that contribute to her well-being. And on other days, she tunes in to a meditation with Dr. Jeffery, during which her silent recitation is "Yes, I am grateful to be alive today."

Brenda admits:

> My past negativities are far away from me. I am only into the now—learning to love me and to love others.

In addition, twice a day, she prioritizes a gratitude tai chi sequence. Before breakfast and again before bed, she rebalances her mind, body and spirit with this practice. Her gratitude routine stretches the hamstrings, the cervical spine, and the lower and upper back as well as toning her calves and thighs.

Sunday is her day of rest and to reconnect. The peaceful Tiger Lady is active with the Bahá'í community while routinely giving thanks to Jesus Christ, who brings her fulfillment.

> As a Tiger Lady, I walk my path, assured of the person I have become—someone who is adaptable and retains deeply rooted values. I am the Tiger Lady who believes nothing is impossible with God.

Brenda Bell's Five Easy Tips

1. Display gratitude with a great attitude.
   Incorporate positive mindfulness practices into your daily routine, like a gratitude journal.

2. Adopt great habits that lead to greater happiness.
   Focus on positivity, smiles, movement and meditation. Choose to be in the company of cheerful, supportive people to keep you going.

3. Take control of your life.
   When you think it's tough, know that God, the Creator, Krishna, Buddha, Allah, whatever name you choose, is on your side. So be true to yourself.

4. Don't give up.
   Grow. Mind over matter. Keep your eye on the prize. Long journeys begin with small steps.

5. Smile, no matter what.
   It makes a difference. Repeat Brenda's mantra: "I smile because it makes me happy. It allows me to be in the moment. In control. Loving. Giving. Compassionate."

The Great Gratitude

I view my life as devoid of suffering; not that I haven't experienced challenges and pains, but I choose to create contentment. Joy is contagious. I frequently visualize the Dalai Lama and his colossal smile. He exudes happiness despite the adversity the Tibetans have endured for generations. Throughout my career, I have known only a few people who radiated positivity, like Brenda. I focus on their smiling faces too.

Brenda suggests surrounding yourself with uplifting people. I first learned about the power of the *sangha* (community of like-minded people) at the Sivananda Yoga Farm (which was discussed in "Chapter 10: Serving is the Secret of Abundance").

I built my sangha little by little from scratch and erected imaginary barriers to the negativity surrounding me. While you cannot live your life in a bubble, you can redirect your time and attention to those who bring more grace into your world.

After time spent with Swami Sita at the Yoga Farm, my lessons continued during the three-hour bus ride to the airport. Images of cherished longtime friends popped up in my head—and heart. It dawned on me that even though they were scattered across the United States, they could be in my sangha. That day, I connected with them from the bus, the airport or as soon as my plane landed. Once home, I vowed to keep these special souls closer, regardless of the distance between us. More than ten years later, I have kept my promise to myself, and my dear, like-minded friends have reciprocated.

Giving thanks every day, I make and hand out gratitude cards to all my students, encouraging them to extend the concept of thanksgiving into a lifestyle. Gratitude messages are like coins in a piggy bank. Stuff that container with thoughts of thankfulness. If you are feeling down, pull a message out to uplift you.

I try to invite gratitude to seep into my life in creative forms. I find most of India Arie's music cheerful and inspiring. A favorite song I play during my yoga classes is Arie's "Give Thanks." The chorus teaches to cherish each day, without waiting for tomorrow. Live in the present and give praise now.

When your work or personal life is bursting with negativity, your first reaction may be to retreat. A gratitude practice should never be intimidating. Actions can be as simple as choosing to read something positive at lunchtime rather than listening to gossip in the lunchroom. It may be going home to unwind instead of hitting the bars, or listening to soothing music instead of watching the nightly news.

Many years ago, when I suffered through bouts of insomnia, I tuned in to the Public Broadcasting Service (PBS) in the middle of the night for a dose of classical music or ballet rather than the in-your-face screaming and fear-producing content that frequented the other channels.

Negativity breeds negativity. Optimism rubs off when gratitude is in the expression, words or movement of another. However, it is possible to repel negativity and attract positivity. Gratitude is a positive magnet and a crucial building block for a healthy soul.

In my experience, Brenda's assertion that smiling is contagious is true. By showing joy to others, the sense of satisfaction becomes magnified and returns to you. Psychologists at the University of Wisconsin explored social mimicry.[141] They determined when someone smiles, you want to do the same. When you see a person cry, you become tearful. The mirror effect is triggered in the orbitofrontal cortex of the brain, which interconnects with the limbic system. This is where emotions rule. There is a clear connection between gratefulness and mental health. Researchers have linked a gratitude practice to a variety of boons, including better moods and sleep patterns.[142]

A happy face is not a mask to hide your gloom. It changes your mood. Smiling increases the neuropeptides in the brain, which are stress eliminators. Dopamine, endorphins and serotonin also kick in, which counteract depression. Endorphins are also pain-relievers.[143] Exercise releases them. You can double the benefits of your workout by grinning.

It is second nature for children to laugh, smile and feel the itch to play and run around. Yet too often adults reach for alcohol or drugs to make themselves feel better, which only makes things worse.

Physical benefits arise from the practice of gratitude too. A collaborative study by psychologists at two universities indicated that those with gratitude journals exercised more and required fewer visits to the doctor.[144] According to a 2018 article from NIH News in Health, Northwestern University researchers found a daily practice of gratitude reduced the incidence of heart disease.[145]

At Berkeley, three hundred adults (mostly students) suffering from anxiety and depression participated in a study on the effectiveness of gratitude. MRI brain imaging confirmed that the gratitude practice subjects displayed greater activity in the medial prefrontal cortex.[146] They felt better because the brain adapted. What's more, those positive effects lingered for several months.

One investigation evaluated Vietnam veterans. Post-traumatic stress syndrome was less common among those with higher levels of gratefulness.[147] Another inquiry identified the positive effects of gratitude following the September 11 traumatic events. The group practicing gratefulness showed greater resiliency.[148] No matter how painful our lives may be, we can all benefit from the effects of giving thanks.

As a holistic health coach, it's clear to me that in our society teeming with trauma, practicing gratitude can kick it in the butt.

||||||||||||||||||||||||||||||||||||||||||||||||||||||||||||||||||||||||||||||||||||||||||||||||||||||||||||||||||||||||||||||||||||||||||||||

Give It a Try:
Daily Gratitude Cards

Get creative. Design your own set of gratitude cards so the images and expressions resonate with you. Find a dozen quotes that inspire you. These could be quotes from within this chapter or from artists or celebrities. For example, Henri Matisse once said, "There are always flowers for those who want to see them."

When you have collected your quotes, lay them out with two, four or six to a page. Pick cheerful font types and colors. For the reverse side, select a pleasing geometric or landscape pattern to fill the entire page. Or incorporate photos of yourself and loved ones. Lay them out to fit the same number per page as you did the quotes. Print them double-sided on card stock and then cut them out. Place the cards in a stack and tie it with a ribbon or yarn.

Every day, pull one from the stack, read the uplifting message, and keep the card with you. Or post the message on your bedroom mirror or refrigerator door. Better yet, share them with your loved ones every day. This is an easy way to begin your journey of practicing gratitude.

Now that you've received the wisdom of my gurus, it's time to assess the teachings that have made a difference in your life and implement new positive habits of your own.

Discovering Your Own Wisdom

*F*rom *the Boxing Ring to the Ashram* provides recipes for becoming more positive, productive and fulfilled, but without having to go through too many hoops to discover how to accomplish that all on your own. Ease into your practices and achievements, then build on them.

The wisdom shared in this book reflects simple and pleasurable practices to help you live right, eat right, love right, and even laugh right. Today, tomorrow and every day, whatever "right" is for you, that is what you need to practice. Listen to your body and intuition. Your regimen is not for anyone else. It is what you choose to enhance your time on earth.

Go at your own pace, but don't be stagnant. When we temporarily stop any routine, it can be difficult to get back on track. Humans thrive on patterns, so stick to one that fits your personal needs.

Some people may prefer to focus on one or two facets of their life for many months. Others might embrace one new practice a month and acquire all twelve habits covered in this book within a year. Maybe you begin with selfless service, and when you're ready, start a gratitude journal. Whatever you do, don't replace the new habit of selfless service with the one of writing in your journal. Rather than swapping or forgetting new behaviors, keep doing what you're doing and add more practices to it.

As you continue your journey, it may be appropriate to recognize those teachers who have already influenced or supported your personal health and well-being.

Identifying Your Gurus

Now that you have explored the teachings of a dozen of my gurus, a good exercise is to reflect upon who your life's greatest teachers are. Maybe it is your parents or another relative, your family physician, a religious or political leader, or a mentor you had at work or school. Take time to acknowledge your inspirations.

Compile a list of six or more people who made an impact in your life. They can still be alive or have already passed on. Jot down what you learned from them and how you put those lessons into practice. Then think of how you can share that wisdom with others. Keep the light, love and lessons of your most cherished teachers shining brightly.

Review your list periodically. Be grateful for the big "G" Gurus or little "g" gurus who helped shape or motivate you. Honor and cherish them. Hold their lessons close to your heart and mind.

Identifying Your Fears and Potential

To get past fears and inhibitions, some adults may find it beneficial to imagine their carefree childhood days. Children have fewer fears when trying something new. They learn to ride a bike by picking themselves up and putting their feet back on the pedals despite scratched knees. Balancing and moving forward becomes smooth sailing with practice. The child wobbling around on a two-wheeler is motivated by the joy and freedom of riding the bike.

Too often, as we grow into adults, our inhibitions increase. We are afraid of criticism and failure. If you've tried diet after diet or to stop smoking time after time, your inner voice may tell you, "Forget it. You can't succeed." Or you're concerned about what your friends or family will say. Many of us have heard throughout our lives, "You can't do that." Wrong!

You can. It's just mind over matter. Shut out the outer criticism and that squeaky, fearful inner voice and begin.

You get to choose the time and place to jump over hurdles, defeat your fears, and change your habits. That decision to act differently comes from within. Seeking help to stop smoking or starting a new diet only works when you are dedicated to making a difference. If you are not committed, the greatest plan will fail. Your willpower and goals are your biggest cheerleaders. A kick in the pants may get you going, but it won't give you the stamina to reach the finish line. Your commitment and determination will take you there.

None of the gurus in this book sailed through life without obstacles. Those dubious detours and stumbling blocks helped guide them to where they are today. They saw their challenges as inspiring.

Your wake-up call might be an automobile accident, distressing lab results, or watching a loved one suffer. But you can preempt the worries and pain. Set your goals now. Find the strength to follow through and fight for positive results.

It's Your Turn

1. Make a list of three personal growth goals.

2. List steps to achieve your goals.

3. Identify and write your compelling reasons for making these changes that will keep you focused.

4. Commit to achieve your goal. Write your affirmations in the present tense.

For example, you may be a diabetic and fear the loss of a limb or other complications. You might want to reduce your reliance on alcohol and electronic devices and become more present in the moment. Your prioritized plan might look like the following:

Goal #1:

Control my diabetes.

Steps:

- Walk thirty minutes a day.
- Change my diet.
- Practice gentle yoga every other day.
- Consult my physician and endocrinologist regularly.

Reasons:

- Live a longer, healthier life.
- Enjoy quality time with my kids and grandkids.
- Minimize the risk of other related health issues.

My affirmation: I control my physical well-being.

Goal #2:

Stop drinking alcohol.

Steps:

- Find a replacement drink, such as flavored sparking water or a sugar-free mocktail.
- Take a brisk walk whenever I feel the urge to reach for

an alcoholic beverage.

- Meditate and practice breathwork routinely.

Reasons:

- Eliminate the negative side effects of alcohol on my blood sugar and my emotional state.
- Have a clearer mind.
- Build self-confidence and interpersonal relationships.

My *affirmation:* I am healthy and happy without alcohol. I find strength in nature's bounty.

Goal #3:

Live in the moment.

Steps:

- Choose a day and time to shut down electronic devices.
- Plan how to fill the time so it isn't boring.
- Seek live events and opportunities to socialize.

Reasons:

- Increase mindfulness and awareness.
- Achieve secondary goals and personal projects that get put aside.
- Be more fulfilled with positive social interaction.

My *affirmation:* I am fulfilled by taking things day by day, enjoying the simple things in life.

Give your commitment the importance it deserves. Don't just scribble the words down on scratch paper. Frame a needle-point rendition of your pledge as a reminder. Design a collage, poster or T-shirt to convey the message. Print your pledge on a pocket-sized reminder encased in plastic and read it every morning. However you choose to celebrate your pledge, keep it somewhere prominent so you will be reminded of it throughout the day.

You don't have to achieve everything at one time. The order in which you pursue your goals may matter. (For example, before coming off antidepressants, you may need to first talk to your psychiatrist, then practice meditation and begin your exercise routine.) The most important thing is committing to the first step.

To help keep you on track, I have created a tracker for you that you can find on my website at deborahcharnes.com/tracker. You can fill that out or create something similar for yourself. Journal your progress on paper or your phone.

If you'd like, you can also join my Facebook group at deborahcharnes.com/fb for virtual check-ins, questions and answers. I also offer monthly virtual retreats for you to take advantage of. They are announced on my website and on Instagram (@deborahcharnes). Plus, you can find many tutorials on my YouTube channel (deborahcharnes.com/youtube).

As you finish reading this book, let me leave you with these parting words.

Live your best life.

Incorporate the wisdom you have learned
into your routines.

Reach for the blessings that are
right there in front of you.

And finally...
Enjoy and share your celebration
of healthy living with others.

The Thirteenth Guru

The one guru missing from this book is my mother. Her physical appearance, personality and emotions seemed to be the opposite of mine. When she wheeled me around in my baby buggy, people questioned whether we were related. Her pitch-black hair and brown eyes did not match my blue eyes and light blond Shirley Temple-like ringlets.

Although the similarities were difficult to recognize before, now I see many shared attributes. Without a doubt, she was my greatest guru, and this book would not exist if not for her.

My mother was a writer. White-out, felt-tipped pens, and colored paper for her drafts cluttered half of the kitchen table. Even after the invention of word processors, she banged everything out on her clunky black upright Royal manual typewriter, striking those keys with force so something would appear on the page. Her reward was a high-pitched "ping" whenever she hit the return key. Before the days of memory chips or cards, every rewrite called for new sheets of paper.

She was tenacious, receiving rejection letter after rejection letter. My dad complained that the earnings for her writing barely covered the postage from her submissions, which were sent by mail with a self-addressed stamped return envelope.

Motivated by fact-finding before the age of Google, Alexa or virtual assistants, she crammed subject-labeled notebooks and big manila envelopes filled with her research into our kitchen cabinets and sometimes called the local librarian to fact-check.

She was creative and resourceful in a quirky way. She *up*cycled before the days of recycling. Dressed in Bermuda shorts and an old button-down shirt, she painted, stained, refinished and reconfigured antique furniture and floor-to-ceiling framed pictures and stacks of tchotchkes.

My mother saw every human as equal. Emma Lazarus's words on the Statue of Liberty, welcoming the tired, the poor and the huddled masses, fueled my mother's commitment to fight for the rights of others in our country and other nations. She lent her voice at assembly halls. She penned hundreds of letters to the editor, earning an award from *The Chicago Tribune*. She carried placards at demonstrations. Once, journalists visited our home to photograph her advocacy in action.

In place of a turban wrapped around her head like some gurus, she hid her thinning hair under a babushka. She always dressed in sky blue, which she said made her feel good. But she taught me to see people beyond their clothing, beyond their material possessions, and beyond society's labels. And these are some of the lessons that drove me to help others by writing this book.

Like my mother, I am down-to-earth, rational and pragmatic. For most of my life, I could not understand the spiritual dimension of existence. With a science-based leaning, it was hard for me to conceptualize the intangible.

Yet I felt compelled to share what took me a lot of time and money to learn. You *can* be your happiest and healthiest. Adapt and adopt my gurus' recommended habits as you feel comfortable to attain a higher quality of physical, emotional or spiritual health. Remember that everything is intertwined: mind, body and spirit. So don't ignore the invisible.

Thank you for reading *From the Boxing Ring to the Ashram*. If you've enjoyed reading this book, please leave a review on your favorite review site. It helps me reach readers who might benefit from the information provided here.

Connect with the Gurus

I hope you've enjoyed getting to know my gurus and exploring the lessons they've taught me. Follow my mentors or learn more about the work they're doing by visiting these sites (in order of their chapters in the book).

- Christopher Perkins – deborahcharnes.com/perkins.
- Dr. Sat Bir Singh Khalsa – deborahcharnes.com/khalsa.
- Lenín Moreno Garcés – deborahcharnes.com/lenin.
- Randall and Kristin Brooks – deborahcharnes.com/brooks.
- Dr. Loren Fishman – deborahcharnes.com/fishman.
- Dr. P. R. Vishnu – deborahcharnes.com/vishnu.
- Chaitanya Charan Das – deborahcharnes.com/chaitanya.
- Rabbi Sarah Schechter – deborahcharnes.com/sarah.
- Gloria Camarillo Vasquez – deborahcharnes.com/gloria.
- Swami Sitaramananda – deborahcharnes.com/sita.
- Radhanath Swami – deborahcharnes.com/radhanath.
- Brenda Bell – deborahcharnes.com/brenda.

And, of course, if you enjoyed this book and would like to connect with me further, I would welcome hearing from you too. You can reach out to me at deborahcharnes.com.

Acknowledgments

First off, I am filled with gratitude to you, the reader. You are the reason I dedicated a significant amount of the last few years to this book. It is my sincerest desire that the teachings from my gurus inspire you to be your healthiest and happiest. Thank you too to the coronavirus. While I'm heartbroken by the coronavirus's devastation, which took so many lives, including those of people I knew, the initial months of lockdown were a breakthrough for me. I spent most of my waking hours in introspection. Inspiration for *From the Boxing Ring to the Ashram* materialized immediately. It was time to honor my gurus and share their simple but effective teachings with the world.

Thank you, Christopher Perkins.

Thank you, Dr. Khalsa.

Thank you, Lenín Moreno.

Thank you, Randall and Kristin Brooks.

Thank you, Dr. Fishman.

Thank you, Dr. Vishnu.

Thank you, Chaitanya Charan Das.

Thank you, Rabbi Sarah Schechter.

Thank you, Gloria Camarillo.

Thank you, Swami Sita.

Thank you, Radhanath Swami.

Thank you, Brenda Bell.

You each inspired countless individuals long before I met you. Your wisdom, methods and approaches forever affected me and my role as a yoga therapist.

Special thanks to my sister, Joanna Charnes. She was my cheerleader throughout the journey. Both she and her son, Jeff Rosenthal, provided on-point direction and feedback when the book was just in the outline stage. My psychotherapist daughter, Viana Vallejo, was also a very level-headed sounding board for elements in Part One.

Early on, I enlisted the editorial aid of Richard Lynch. I'm grateful that he never stopped pushing me to refine my content.

After umpteen sets of revisions, I completed the manuscript. I manifested for a professional, passionate publishing partner— for a long time. I became discouraged. Was I not manifesting correctly? Were my vision boards not clear?

Fortunately, fellow yoga therapist and author of *Enlighten Up* and *Soul Food*, Beth Gibbs, directed me to Emerald Lake Books.

From the first Emerald Lake Books YouTube video I watched, I knew publisher Tara Alemany was who I needed. She was exactly what I had been manifesting. Tara has become my business coach, editor, literary guru and passionate professional partner. I can't thank her enough, nor can I imagine repeating the process without her.

Tara's partner, Mark Gerber, was a wonderful sounding board and, most importantly, he seemed to totally "get" me and how I wanted to convey my book. His design layouts were spot on. Oddly enough, after viewing the proposed cover art, I pulled one of Radhanath Swami's oracle cards. The image and message were suggestive of Mark's creative concept.

Finally, I give eternal thanks to my mom. She taught me about grammar and style as well as persistence, compassion and altruism.

About the Author

R iddled with chronic lower back pain and digestive disorders since childhood, Deborah Charnes spent fifty years exploring the world, uncovering secrets to health and happiness.

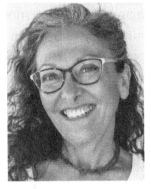

For two decades, she managed hundreds of news conferences, editorial board meetings, press briefings, and one-on-one interviews. She worked with security, communications and advance teams for John McCain, Hillary Clinton, President Barack Obama, First Lady Michelle Obama, then-Vice President Joe Biden, Dr. Jill Biden, Bernie Sanders, megastar Jennifer Lopez, and the Vice President of El Salvador.

To balance the chaotic scales directing major league campaigns, it was essential for her to soothe the stress and 24/7 schedule with body, mind and spirit lifesavers.

In 2011, Deborah left the high-pressure demands as an international corporate marketing communications strategist. Moving forward, she dedicated that same energy to positive transformation—of herself and others. She vowed to never stop learning—or sharing.

Deborah has published more than five hundred mind/body and lifestyle articles, and in 2021, she joined AARP's The Ethel as a contributing writer.

Already a certified yoga teacher, she added training in Ayurvedic massage therapy, nutrition and cooking. She received certification in yin, restorative and yoga nidra therapies, acupressure and reiki, and became one of the first bilingual (English/Spanish) certified yoga therapists in Texas.

Coaching people of all ages all over the world and with many physical or emotional challenges, she seeks to boost the mind, body and spirit through simple techniques that can be practiced anywhere and anytime. To that end, she has created many signature therapeutic workshops and offers Wisdom Weekend retreats. You can view her current offerings on her website at deborahcharnes.com.

When not writing, traveling or working with her yoga students and therapy clients, Deborah enjoys hosting guests at her mini retreat center, The Namaste Getaway, in Texas Hill Country. If you're interested in booking one-on-one yoga therapy or a therapeutic getaway with her, visit deborahcharnes.com/getaway.

If you're interested in having Deborah speak to your group or organization, you can contact her at emeraldlakebooks.com/charnes.

Notes

Lessons for Unlikely Gurus
1   The American Association of Retired Persons is an organization that focuses on issues affecting those over the age of fifty.
2   Sivananda, Swami, *Bliss Divine*. Divine Life Society, Rishikesh, India, 1951.

Chapter I
3   Traditional call-and-response meditational chants.
4   A Native American rite of passage that typically entails meditative solitary periods in nature, where one has to fend for oneself.
5   The Ayurvedic constitution associated with air and ether, frequently manifested by a highly active body or mind.
6   The repetition of a set number of syllables, usually a short prayer or affirmation, which calms the mind. It can be in any language, but within the yogic communities, Sanskrit or Gurmukhi mantras are common.
7   "What is imagery?" Johns Hopkins Medicine. Accessed Apr 15, 2023. deborahcharnes.com/hopkinsmedicine.
8   Luders, Eileen et al. "The unique brain anatomy of meditation practitioners: alterations in cortical gyrification." *Frontiers in human neuroscience*, vol. 6:34, Feb 29, 2012. doi:10.3389/fnhum.2012.00034.
9   "Former Surgeon General Discusses Stress and Well-Being at 2017 Straus Lecture." *National Center for Complementary and Integrative Health*, Sept 21, 2017. deborahcharnes.com/vivek.

10   Sage, Laura. "Six Proven Benefits of Meditation in the Workplace." *Forbes*, Jul 31, 2020. deborahcharnes.com/workplace.

11   Fell, Andy. "Mindfulness from meditation associated with lower stress hormone," *UCDavis*, Mar 27, 2013. deborahcharnes.com/stresshormone.

12   For more information, visit deborahcharnes.com/breathing.

13   There is no actual meaning to the letters O and M. However, they are sacred sounds. Om is a seed mantra or celestial sound that contains multiple sounds and vibrations.

14   The sanskrit word for "peace."

Chapter 2

15   A three-string, long-necked musical instrument that dates back to the 16th century in central Asia. Ravi Shankar introduced the music of the sitar to the West at the 1971 Concert for Bangladesh he organized with George Harrison of the Beatles.

16   The subtitle tells it all. "From Emerson and the Beatles to Yoga and Meditation; How Indian Spirituality Changed the West."

17   "Post-Traumatic Stress Disorder (PTSD) 2022," *National Institutes of Health*. Accessed Apr 15, 2023. deborahcharnes.com/ptsd.

18   "How Common is PTSD in Adults?" *US Department of Veterans Affairs*. Accessed Apr 15, 2023. deborahcharnes.com/vaptsd.

19   A form of psychotherapy designed to help people respond in more positive ways to stress, negative situations or thoughts.

20   Jindani, Farah et al. "A Yoga Intervention for Posttraumatic Stress: A Preliminary Randomized Control Trial." Evidence-based complementary and alternative medicine : eCAM vol. 2015 (2015): 351746. Aug 20, 2015. doi:10.1155/2015/351746.

21   Johnston, Jennifer M. et al. "Yoga for military service personnel with PTSD: A single arm study." *Psychological trauma: theory, research, practice and policy* vol. 7,6 (2015): 555-62. doi:10.1037/tra0000051.

22   Descilo, T. et al. "Effects of a yoga breath intervention alone and in combination with an exposure therapy for post-traumatic stress disorder and depression in survivors of the 2004 South-East Asia tsunami." *Acta Psychiatrica Scandinavica* vol. 121,4 (2010): 289-300. doi:10.1111/j.1600-0447.2009.01466.x.

23   "Depressive Disorder (Depression)." *World Health Organization*, Mar 31, 2023. deborahcharnes.com/depression.

24   Banov, Dr. Michael. "Is Depression Different in Men and Women?" *Psych Congress Network*, Oct 21, 2022. deborahcharnes.com/genderdepression.

25   "Baby Blues," *American Pregnancy Association*. Accessed April 15, 2023. deborahcharnes.com/babyblues.

26   "Do I Have Baby Blues or Postpartum Depression?" *American Pregnancy Association*. Accessed Apr 15, 2023. deborahcharnes.com/postpartum.

27   At times, brooding thoughts of suicide can accompany depression. Those contemplating suicide or who already have suicidal tendencies should seek immediate help from a mental health professional or, in the United States, call the National Suicide Prevention Lifeline at 988.

28   A class focused on centering and relaxing in each pose rather than creating a more dynamic flow.

29   A form of hatha yoga that focuses on proper alignment.

30   Streeter, Chris C. et al. "Effects of yoga versus walking on mood, anxiety, and brain GABA levels: a randomized controlled MRS study." *Journal of alternative and complementary medicine* (New York, NY) vol. 16,11 (2010): 1145-52. doi:10.1089/acm.2010.0007.

31   Cahn, B. Rael et al. "Yoga, Meditation and Mind-Body Health: Increased BDNF, Cortisol Awakening Response, and Altered Inflammatory Marker Expression after a 3-Month Yoga and Meditation Retreat." *Frontiers in human neuroscience* vol. 11:315. Jun 26, 2017. doi:10.3389/fnhum.2017.00315.

32   Boccia, Maddalena et al. "The Meditative Mind: A Comprehensive Meta-Analysis of MRI Studies." *BioMed research international*, vol. 2015 (2015): 419808. doi:10.1155/2015/419808.

33   A guided meditation that induces a nourishing sleep-like state.

Chapter 3

34   "Vicepresidente condecoró a Patch Adams." *El Universo*, Jun 1, 2007. deborahcharnes.com/patch.

35   Portrayed by Robin Williams in the movie, *Patch Adams*.

36   See footnote 34.

37   Cultura, Redacción. "Lenín Moreno Es El Hombre Del Humor De Resistencia (Video)." *El Telégrafo*, Sep 19, 2014. deborahcharnes.com/humoraward.

38   See note 37.

39   See note 37.

40   Not recommended for people recovering from surgery, pregnant women in the third trimester, or people with angina pain, hernias, epilepsy, incontinence or schizophrenia.

41   "Endorphins: The brain's natural pain reliever," *Harvard Health Publishing*, Jul 20, 2021. deborahcharnes.com/endorphins.

42   Berk, Lee S. et al. "Modulation of Neuroimmune Parameters During the Eustress of Humor-Associated Mirthful Laugher," *Alternative Therapies*, Vol. 7, No. 2, Mar 2001. deborahcharnes.com/goodmedicine.

43   American Physiological Society. "Laughter Remains Good Medicine." *ScienceDaily*, Apr 17, 2009. deborahcharnes.com/laughter.

44   van der Wal, C. Natalie, and Robin N. Kok. "Laughter-inducing therapies: Systematic review and meta-analysis." *Social science & medicine* (1982) vol. 232 (2019): 473-488. doi:10.1016/j.socscimed.2019.02.018.

Chapter 4

45   A portable instrument featuring piano-like keys and accordion-like valves to produce sound. Sometimes called a "pump organ," it is European in origin. During the mid-1800s, in India, the device was modified to make it more portable. Today, it is one of the primary instruments for kirtan.

46   The people in the Indo-Pakistani region that followed Vedic rules were called "Hindus" by the British, which was a variant of the word "Indian." Since it was not self-ascribed, some may choose not to use that word for self-identification.

47   Those who praise Vishnu as the supreme lord. In practice, it extends to those who honor Vishnu's incarnations of Krishna and Rama, as well as their consorts, Radhe and Sita. It is a subset of Hinduism.

48   A religious and philosophical tradition originating in ancient India that emphasizes nonviolence and individual spiritual progress.

49   Martin Luther King, Jr. *Strength to Love*, Harper & Row, 1963.

50   A revered sage and author from the Indian subcontinent who died circa 150 BC. He wrote many Vedic treatises, among which was the *Yoga Sutras*, the bible for yogis.

51   Campbell, Don. *The Mozart Effect*, Quill, Sep 18, 2001.

52   Vickhoff, Björn et al. "Music structure determines heart rate variability of singers." *Frontiers in psychology* vol. 4 334. Jul 9, 2013. doi:10.3389/fpsyg.2013.00334.

53   Bernardi, L. et al. "Effect of rosary prayer and yoga mantras on autonomic cardiovascular rhythms: comparative study." *BMJ (Clinical research ed.)* vol. 323,7327 (2001): 1446-9. doi:10.1136/bmj.323.7327.1446.

Chapter 5

54   An adjective referring to something related to the *Vedas*, the ancient scriptures from the Indian subcontinent.

55   "New Approach Uses Yoga To Help With Rotator Cuff Injuries," CBS *New York*, Jul 2, 2019. deborahcharnes.com/rotatorcuff.

56   International Osteoporosis Foundation. Accessed Apr 15, 2023. deborahcharnes.com/osteoporosis.

57   Lu, Yi-Hsueh et al. "Twelve-Minute Daily Yoga Regimen Reverses Osteoporotic Bone Loss." Topics in geriatric rehabilitation vol. 32,2 (2016): 81-87. doi:10.1097/tgr.0000000000000085.

58   "Loren Fishman," *Omega*. Accessed Apr 11, 2023. deborahcharnes.com/fishmanbio.

59   Sri is an honorary title, similar to "Master" or "Sir."

60   Krishnamacharya is often considered the father of modern yoga. In addition, his teachings influence today's yoga therapy profession.

61   Smith, Laura. "39 Global Back Pain Statistics: How Common is Back Pain?" *The Good Body*, No 14, 2022. deborahcharnes.com/backpain.

62   Lucas, Jacqueline W. et al. "Back, Lower Limb, and Upper Limb Pain Among US Adults, 2019," Centers for Disease Control and Prevention, NCHS *Data Brief*, no. 415, Jul 2021. deborahcharnes.com/paincomplaint.

63   "US National Survey Identifies Associations Between Chronic Severe Back Pain and Disability," *National Institutes of Health*, Sep 9, 2022. deborahcharnes.com/disability.

64   Fiorenzi, Ryan. "23 Back Pain Statistics and Facts That Will Surprise You." *Start Standing*, Jan 15, 2023. deborahcharnes.com/opioids.

65   "Drug Overdose Deaths Remain High." Centers for Disease Control and Prevention, *Death Rate Maps and Graphs*, Jun 2, 2022. deborahcharnes.com/overdose.

66   Meran, Daniel, MD. "10 Reasons for a visit to your primary care physician." *Detroit Free Press*, Apr 29, 2022. deborahcharnes.com/doctorvisits.

67   Sheng, Jiyao et al. "The Link between Depression and Chronic Pain: Neural Mechanisms in the Brain." *Neural plasticity* vol. 2017 (2017): 9724371. doi:10.1155/2017/9724371.

68   A narrowing of the spinal canal causing pressure on the spinal cord and nerve roots.

69   A condition where one of the vertebrae slips, causing pressure on a nerve.

70   A condition where muscles press against the sciatic nerve.

71   The state where the spine has rounding at the thoracic area (upper back). In olden days, extreme cases were referred to as "hunchback" or "dowager's hump."

72   Unlike kyphosis, this anatomical variance is when there is a pronounced arch in the lower back and often a tilting forward of the pelvis.

73   For more information about this pose, visit deborahcharnes.com/sphinx.

74   For more information about this pose, visit deborahcharnes.com/fish.

75   For more information about this pose, visit deborahcharnes.com/bridge.

76   For more information about this pose, visit deborahcharnes.com/plank.

77   For more information about this sequence of poses, visit deborahcharnes.com/sunsalutation.

78   For more information about this pose, visit deborahcharnes.com/lordofthefish.

79   For more information about this pose, visit deborahcharnes.com/twistedtriangle.

80   For more information about this pose, visit deborahcharnes.com/boat.

81   For more information about this pose, visit deborahcharnes.com/forwardfold.

82   For more information about this pose, visit deborahcharnes.com/childspose.

83   Zou, Liye et al. "Are Mindful Exercises Safe and Beneficial for Treating Chronic Lower Back Pain? A Systematic Review and

Meta-Analysis of Randomized Controlled Trials." *Journal of clinical medicine* vol. 8,5 628. May 8, 2019. doi:10.3390/jcm8050628.

84   Crow, Edith Meszaros et al. "Effectiveness of Iyengar yoga in treating spinal (back and neck) pain: A systematic review." International journal of yoga vol. 8,1 (2015): 3-14. doi:10.4103/0973-6131.146046.

85   Highland, Krista Beth et al. "Benefits of the Restorative Exercise and Strength Training for Operational Resilience and Excellence Yoga Program for Chronic Low Back Pain in Service Members: A Pilot Randomized Controlled Trial." *Archives of Physical Medicine and Rehabilitation,* vol. 99, no. 1, Jan 1, 2018, pp. 91–98, doi:10.1016/j.apmr.2017.08.473.

86   For more information about this pose, visit deborahcharnes.com/sixdirections.

Chapter 6

87   Ayurveda teaches that everyone is created with a unique constitution based on a combination of three energetic forces or bodily humors: vata, pitta, and kapha. Wellness involves bringing about the natural state of balance among those constitutions.

88   See footnote 5.

89   The Ayurvedic constitution associated with fire correlates to healthy digestion, among other things.

90   The Ayurvedic constitution associated with earth and water correlates to stability and strength, among other things.

91   "India Ayurvedic Products Market: Industry Trends, Share, Size, Growth, Opportunity and Forecast 2023-2028," IMARC Group. Accessed Apr 12, 2023. deborahcharnes.com/producttrends.

92   Yoga and Ayurveda teach that there are three gunas, qualities or attributes that can cause imbalances. *Rajas,* which is overly passionate, hyperactive, erratic and unnerving. *Tamas,* which is apathetic, lethargic or toxic. And *sattva,* which is considered positive, pure and healthy. Ayurveda and yoga can help keep the guna centered in sattva.

93   "Poor Nutrition." Centers for Disease Control and Prevention, *National Center for Chronic Disease Prevention and Health Promotion,* Sep 8, 2022. deborahcharnes.com/nutrition.

94   "Sodium in your diet," US Food and Drug Administration, Feb 25, 2022. deborahcharnes.com/sodium.

95   "State of Obesity 2022: Better Policies for a Healthier America." *Trust for America's Health,* Sep 27, 2022. deborahcharnes.com/obesity.

96 "Prediabetes – Your Chance to Prevent Type 2 Diabetes." Centers for Disease Control and Prevention, Dec 30, 2022.
deborahcharnes.com/prediabetes.

97 "Chronic Diseases in America." Centers for Disease Control and
Prevention, Dec 13, 2022. deborahcharnes.com/chronicdisease.

98 Sperber, Ami D et al. "Worldwide Prevalence and Burden of
Functional Gastrointestinal Disorders, Results of Rome Foundation Global Study." *Gastroenterology Journal*, Apr 12, 2020.
doi:10.1053/j.gastro.2020.04.014.

99 Byadgi, P. S. et al. "Clinical Assessment of Strength of Agni."
International Journal of Research in Ayurveda & Pharmacy, Dec 14, 2011.
deborahcharnes.com/agni.

100 Guglielmi, Giorgia. "How Many Genes Make up the Human
Microbiome?" *MicrobiomePost*, Clorofilla Srl., Sep 23, 2019.
deborahcharnes.com/microbiome.

101 Steer, Eliot. "A cross comparison between Ayurvedic etiology of
Major Depressive Disorder and bidirectional effect of gut dysregulation." *Journal of Ayurveda and Integrative Medicine* vol. 10, 1 (2019): 59-66.
doi:10.1016/j.jaim.2017.08.002.

Chapter 7

102 "Are there any logical reasons to choose vegetarianism?" The Spiritual Scientist, Jan 13, 2012. deborahcharnes.com/help.

103 People who abstain from eating all animal products, including
dairy, eggs and honey.

104 "Protein: Power Up With Plant-Based Protein." *Physicians Committee for Responsible Medicine*. Accessed Apr 18, 2023.
deborahcharnes.com/protein.

105 "Nutrition and athletic performance," MedlinePlus. Accessed
Apr 18, 2023. deborahcharnes.com/performance.

106 Pachauri, R. K. "Global Warning! The Impact of Meat Production and Consumption on Climate Change." IPCC, Sep 8, 2008.
deborahcharnes.com/meatimpact.

107 FAO, IFAD, UNICEF, WFP and WHO. *The State of Food Security
and Nutrition in the World 2020*. Rome, FAO. Last updated Oct 15, 2021.
doi:10.4060/ca9692en.

108 Kakaei, Hojatollah et al. "Chapter One – Effect of COVID-19
on food security, hunger, and food crisis." COVID-19 and the

Sustainable Development Goals (2022): 3–29. Jul 29, 2022. doi:10.1016/B978-0-323-91307-2.00005-5.

109 Henao, Luis Andres, and Jessie Wardarski. "A Family Struggle as Pandemic Worsens Food Insecurity." *Toronto Star*, Toronto Star Newspapers Ltd., Sep 14, 2020. deborahcharnes.com/foodinsecurity.

110 Pimentel, David and Marcia Pimentel. "Sustainability of meat-based and plant-based diets and the environment," *Am J Clin Nutr* 2003; 78(suppl): 660S–3S. deborahcharnes.com/pimentel.

111 Obama, Michelle. *The Story of the White House Kitchen Garden and Gardens Across America*, Crown, 2012.

112 Robinson, Elizabeth et al. "Spirituality Increases as Alcoholics Recover." *Journal of Studies on Alcohol and Drugs*, vol. 68, no. 2, Mar 2007, pp. 282–290. deborahcharnes.com/sobriety.

113 Chopra, Deepak and Rudolph E. Tanzi. *The Healing Self*, Harmony, 2020.

114 Chopra, Deepak. "The Fatal Prescription Pad." *San Francisco Chronicle*, Dec 14, 2009. deborahcharnes.com/prescriptions.

Chapter 8

115 Also referred to as "the Sabbath."

116 Riedel, Alexander W., "Air Force rabbi 'one of a kind,'" *Air Force News Service*, Apr 4, 2013. deborahcharnes.com/airforcerabbi.

117 US Air Force Recruiting, "US Air Force: Rabbi Sarah Schechter, Jewish Chaplain," YouTube, Dec 29, 2015. deborahcharnes.com/rabbimsg.

118 A paraphrasing of Genesis 2:2b.

119 Michaels, Irene. "Unplugging: A Phenomenological Study of the Perceived Holistic Health Benefits from Regular Digital Detox in the Context of Jewish Shabbat." St. Catherine University, May 2016. deborahcharnes.com/sophia.

120 See note 119.

121 "The Loneliness Epidemic Persists: A Post-Pandemic Look at the State of Loneliness among US Adults," The Cigna Group. Accessed Apr 18, 2023. deborahcharnes.com/loneliness.

122 "Digital Detox." *American Academy of Ophthalmology*. Accessed Apr 18, 2023. deborahcharnes.com/detox.

123 Speedling, B. B. "Celebrating Sabbath as a Holistic Health Practice: The Transformative Power of a Sanctuary in Time." *J Relig Health* 58, 1382–1400 (2019). doi:10.1007/s10943-019-00799-6.

Chapter 9

124 A fresh dough made from maize (corn).

125 Indigenous people from central Mexico.

126 A South American tree otherwise known as "holy wood." While sage is believed to clear out negativity, palo santo is thought to bring back the good.

127 A female faith-healer or woman well-versed in blessings, potions and natural remedies.

128 Nautiyal, Chandra Shekhar et al. "Medicinal smoke reduces airborne bacteria." *Journal of ethnopharmacology* vol. 114,3 (2007): 446-51. doi:10.1016/j.jep.2007.08.038.

129 Federation of American Societies for Experimental Biology. "Burning incense is psychoactive: New class of antidepressants might be right under our noses." ScienceDaily, May 20, 2008. deborahcharnes.com/incense.

Chapter 10

130 Inspired by Swami Sivananda Saraswati, who established his first ashram in 1932 in Rishikesh, India.

131 Sivananda Yoga Farm. "Swami Sitaramananda Presenting Herself." YouTube, Mar 27, 2013. deborahcharnes.com/swamisita.

132 Sivananda Yoga Farm. "Karma Yoga: What Is Action in Inaction and Inaction in Action?" YouTube, Jun 28, 2020. deborahcharnes.com/karmayoga.

133 Sitaramananda, Swami. "The Yoga of Selflessness." *Sivananda Yoga Farm*, Apr 16, 2014. deborahcharnes.com/selflessness.

134 Kumar, Arun, and Sanjay Kumar. "Karma yoga: A path towards work in positive psychology." *Indian journal of psychiatry*, vol. 55 (Suppl 2): pp S150-2, Jan 2013. doi:10.4103/0019-5545.105511.

135 Navare, A., and Pandey, A. "Karma Yoga: Scale development and studies of the impact on positive psychological outcomes at the workplace." *International Journal of Cross Cultural Management*, 22(2), 271–299, Jul 11, 2022. doi:/10.1177/14705958221111239.

136 Johnson, John A. "Selfless Service, Part I: Is Selfless Service Possible?" *Psychology Today*, Sussex Publishers, May 8, 2013. deborahcharnes.com/selflessservice.

Chapter 11

137 In 1965, at the age of sixty-nine, Srila Prabhupada left India on a cargo ship with just a few dollars. Within twelve years, he established 108 Krishna temples, ashrams, schools and farm communities. As an author, his books have been translated into seventy-six languages.

138 Contentment is one of the ten principles from Patanjali's Yoga Sutras, similar to the Ten Commandments, referred to in the Sutras as santosha.

139 Dunn, Elizabeth W. et al. "If money doesn't make you happy, then you probably aren't spending it right." *Journal of Consumer Psychology*, 21(2), 115–125, Mar 21, 2011. doi:10.1016/j.jcps.2011.02.002.

140 Donnelly, Grant E. et al. "The Amount and Source of Millionaires' Wealth (Moderately) Predict Their Happiness." *Personality and Social Psychology Bulletin*, 44(5), 684–699, Jan 11, 2018. doi:10.1177/0146167217744766.

Chapter 12

141 Gray, Richard. "It's not just yawning—smiling and frowning are contagious too! We mimic other people's expressions to show empathy," *Daily Mail*, Feb 11, 2016. deborahcharnes.com/socialmimicry.

142 Mills, Paul J. et al. "The Role of Gratitude in Spiritual Well-being in Asymptomatic Heart Failure Patients." *Spirituality in clinical practice (Washington, DC)*, 2(1), 5–17, 2015. doi:10.1037/scp0000050.

143 "Health Benefits of Smiling," Narayana Health, Oct 7, 2022. deborahcharnes.com/smiling.

144 "Practicing Gratitude." *National Institutes of Health*, Jul 25, 2022. deborahcharnes.com/gratitude.

145 "Giving Thanks Can Make You Happier." *Harvard Health Publishing*, Aug 14, 2021. deborahcharnes.com/givingthanks.

146 Brown, Joshua, and Joel Wong. "How Gratitude Changes You and Your Brain." *Greater Good Magazine*, Jun 6, 2017. deborahcharnes.com/gratitudeeffect.

147 Adkins, Clara I. "Improving Veterans' Psychological Well-Being with a Positive Psychology Gratitude Exercise" Doctor of Philosophy (PhD), Dissertation, Counseling and Human Services, Old Dominion University, December 2020. doi:10.25777/vmb6-ph75.

148 Hampton, Tiffanie. "Give Gratitude a Shot," Texas Military Department, Nov 1, 2018. deborahcharnes.com/gratitudeshot.

For more great books, please visit us at
emeraldlakebooks.com.

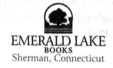

EMERALD LAKE
BOOKS
Sherman, Connecticut